ReStart

Burnout Recovery from a Patient Perspective

Rogier van Kralingen

©Rogier van Kralingen 2018
All Rights Reserved
Publisher INNOA Amsterdam / TheWholeStory
Editor Carolyn Nelson
Cover design Martijn Lap / Mercl.com
ISBN Number 9789082331035
www.restart-burnout-book.com
After an idea from TheWholeStory
www.thewholestory.eu

For Brigitte, who gave me a restart in more ways than I could have ever imagined.

My Help Team

Thanks to my mother, father and brother for just letting me be. My old friend Dr. Metten Somers (PhD) for helping me understand what I was going through. To Lauren Verster, Sandra Lewitz and Anne Schipper, all three for the same reason: we help each other through tough times - always. To my general practitioner dr. Hezemans. To my old buddy Martijn van der Schouw and my new buddy Erik Hopman for the chiropractics and physiotherapy. To Martijn Lap for the cover, as ever you are my creative master. To Wouter van Ewijk for his invaluable advice. To Kerim Fathallah for strengthening me with mindfulness. To Djilani Sprang-Purperhart for his excellent coaching. To Ralph Smart for his positive video's. To Jan Volmer for the physical and mental training. And last but definitely not least, a big thanks to haptonomist Carolien van Dijk, who got me back on my feet and inspired me to reach out to the world around me.

And my deepest love and thanks goes to Brigitte Kalkhoven, she knows why.

I wrote this book for all of you, as much as for all the people reading it now.

From the bottom of my heart,

Thank you

Join us at www.restart-burnout-book.com
In this book, we will be exploring signals, triggers, symptoms and causes of burnout, and related conditions such as depression, breakdowns, grief and trauma. The main premise of this book is the Patient Perspective - recognizing that everyone's burnout is unique and finding the solution that works best is just as personal.

You are also invited to explore even more possibilities at www.restart-burnout-book.com where you can read about other people's recovery experiences and share your own. The stories and solutions you share can be edited in revisions of this book, making it a live document with your contributions at the centre.

Together we can help each other!

Introduction

Dear Reader

What you are about to read is a twist on the usual perspective of the burnout phenomenon. I had a lot of help recovering and I have succeeded. Instead of a problem, my burnout turned out to be an opportunity.

But during my recovery journey, there were many important insights missing that I believe would have helped me recover faster. Because I know what you are going through, I would like to share them with you. That's why I have written this book - so you can recover more quickly than I did.

As someone who has been there, I also know you are probably all over the place right now. So we need to get down to ground zero first. Right here, right now, this instant, you need to understand you are not alone. We are in this together. You need to get help from everyone around you - including professionals - and bring together your Help Team immediately. If you haven't done this already, you need to put down this book, grab your phone and call *everyone* who can help.

Done calling? Still here? Good. Then let's get one thing straight: I'm no burnout guru and have no intention of becoming one. I'm just a writer and musician who suffered from what could be called a double burnout: depression and extreme fatigue mixed with a good healthy dose of general anxiety disorder, topped off with a pinch of panic attacks for good measure. I'm a fellow victim, a 'patient' like you. I'm here to be part of your Help Team.

Nothing more, nothing less.

You should know I have fully recovered. I've actually become stronger and healthier than I've ever been. In a sense, I've become whole. I feel truly *free* these days - free of depression and fatigue, my anxiety is manageable and I feel free to do with my life what I want to do.

So although this book should only be seen as supportive to your process, I believe I will be able to give you lots of insight from the patient perspective on what can and will work for your recovery.

Again, you are not alone. There are millions and millions of people who are or have been in a similar situation. Know that your signals, triggers, symptoms, causes and solutions will be highly unique to you. With this book I hope to give you a good grasp of all the tools available to you for a speedy recovery.

Since I have tried a lot of things to get better, I hope sharing my experience with you will help fast forward your recovery. And let me tell you, from breathing in the scent of lavender flowers (which works surprisingly well!) to talking to a psychologist, and from listening to brainwave beats to taking medicine, I have experimented with a lot of different things!

I eventually found my personal key to recovery. With this book, I hope I can help you find your personal key faster and easier than I did. I want to unlock doors that can help you transform your breakdown from a terrifying experience into a golden opportunity to heal and empower yourself.

Welcome to your restart!

Part I: Your Personal Approach

The Perspective I Was Missing

As I said earlier, I had a lot of help in recovering and I am grateful to all the people who helped me get there. But I was missing out on some things that I wished I had known about earlier. I'm going to be sharing all of my experiences with you and I'd like to start with a few insights that you might not find elsewhere.

The first thing I missed was this: I rarely encountered people, lessons or insights that focussed on the emotional grind of burnout or how excruciating the experience itself is. I kept running into websites, books or people giving me guidance. The advice was very welcome of course, but because it never truly considered the emotional turmoil I was in, it also felt as if I was only getting half the story.

They all meant well, and I knew I was going to be ok, just like you already know you will recover. But that's not my point. During the burnout, I needed someone to connect with me on the terrible emotions I was feeling *at that time*. Someone who just shared this feeling and would tell me: this sucks. Basically, someone who would be miserable with me for a while, without offering me help and advice. I craved to just *be*.

Another thing I missed was clarity about the finish line - that you will come out reborn. Make no mistake. You will feel like a phoenix that rises again or a beautiful butterfly that emerges from its cocoon when you recover: the transformation hurts like hell but the result is magnificent.

I needed someone to tell me this whole bloody burnout thing is an opportunity as much as it is a problem. You feel miserable now, which you'll learn is actually fine. But know that eventually, you will feel reborn.

Something else I missed during my burnout was a crystal clear distinction between signals, triggers, symptoms, causes and solutions. Of course it is very likely all sorts of underlying emotions, relations, circumstances and thought processes are at the root of your burnout. You will need to work hard and long on fixing those, but despite what your Help Team will tell you, they might not necessarily be the answer to recovering from your burnout. They could be and often are, so pay attention to them. Just remember that the answer for your recovery is not written in stone.

It could be you will recover by simply learning how to belly breathe, or learning to cope with certain triggers. Or perhaps you will snap out of it by simply understanding the processes of stress building up in your body. None of that excuses you from digging deep and finding the causes of your burnout. Just keep in mind, the way *into* your burnout might only be half of what you need to know in order to get *out* of it.

Also, despite calling ourselves 'patients', what we are concerned with here are treatments, not cures. That's another important insight. You're not sick or going crazy, and you won't be depressed, tired or anxious forever. So you don't need a 'cure'. But you do require a period of treatment, rewiring yourself to better cope with stress, anxiety and negative thoughts and emotions. You give yourself time to restart. I guess that's your cure: time.

In short, that's the story few people will tell you. And that's precisely why it's the story you need to hear. The story from the patient's perspective - the whole story.

Your Personal Approach

The central theme of this book will be the difference between five things: signals, triggers, symptoms, causes and solutions surrounding your burnout. How these five things impact you will be unique – no one person is the same here - so I want to provide you with lots and lots of options to think about and experiment with.

I cannot stress enough how important it will be to make your approach to your recovery a deeply personal one. Why? Well, although it is fast becoming the modern worlds' number one health affliction, to this day there is no solid clinical definition of burnout in existence. It's just a general term that encompasses everything from fried nerves to depression to anxiety disorders coupled with both physical and mental breakdowns.

So there you go. You have an affliction that doctors haven't been able to define! Great... That's why there is no 'cure' and no such thing as a 'program' that works for everyone. Yet, you *are* burned out and I gather that if you bought this book you'd like to recover from that!

Have no fear. This is the very reason I wrote this book. The fact that there is no solid definition also means that the only approach that will work for you will have to be tailor made. That is actually very good news. I can tell you from experience that the more personal your approach, the better. To emphasize this, I'm going to illustrate a couple of examples that show just how personal a recovery can be.

Some people will find that talking about their deepest emotional distress will help them recover. But for others, the key to recovery might lie in their diet. Still another person might have to deal with anxiety triggers before the burnout subsides. And some of you will have to quit your job or change a relationship you're in before you recover.

There are people out there who will need to do all of the above and much more. People who will need to change their lives completely and work on their issues and recovery for years. But there are also people reading this who just need to learn how to belly breathe. And *poof*, these feelings of burnout will be gone.

Are you catching my drift? This what I mean with the patients' perspective in the subtitle of the book: despite what many people, including professional helpers will say, your burnout and your recovery are *highly personal*. Again, the more personalized your approach, the faster you will recover.

Let me show you what I mean by telling you part of my own story. For me to recover from my depression and general fatigue, it was very important I talked about my deepest feelings. I needed to get to the *cause* of things and dig very deep within myself. It was a process that took me a very long time, drained me and made me extremely vulnerable.

In that vulnerable period, I became more susceptible to anxiety than ever. Through some cruel twist of fate, I developed a general anxiety disorder during that time. So on top of feeling depressed from all the emotional digging I'd been doing, I also suffered from regular panic attacks. In fact, even later when my whole life had changed for the better and I had basically recovered from my burnout... I still had panic attacks.

My Help Team urged me to get to the deepest causes of this as well. They pushed me to go deeper and deeper into my worst fears. So in I went again. But while facing those fears was really helpful to me as a person, it didn't actually relieve my anxiety. Not in the slightest. I was left having faced all my fears – from the smallest to biggest - but continued to suffer from panic attacks.

To recover from the anxiety disorder, I discovered that I just needed to learn how the so-called 'panic trick' works and what you can do about it. I needed to know about *triggers and symptoms*. Including how to restore a faulty breathing pattern. The solution to the panic attacks had literally nothing to do with the *causes* of my burnout.

Zilch.

(Note: For those of you suffering from panic attacks, please have a look at the Extra's section at the end of this book where I cover this topic in greater depth.)

This is essentially what I have learned: going *into* a burnout is different from getting *out*, and the solution to burnout is always highly personal. So let's dedicate a page to clearly state the differences between five aspects of burnout.

Signals, Triggers, Symptoms, Causes & Solutions

Signals – With signals we mean emotions that flow through you. A signal could be that you feel uncomfortable, fearful or irritated, perhaps in a crowd, at work or when you meet a specific person. Signals start mostly in the subconscious mind. Learning to recognize and be mindful of them will help you recover.

Triggers – Triggers are the things that spur you into action or inaction based on the emotional signals you feel. Triggers can be things like loud noises, traffic or even food. They happen to you, coincide with what you feel and then make you either do something or not.

Symptoms – Symptoms are formed from the triggers that lead you to act or not act, and can best be described as the physical manifestations such as shortness of breath, headaches, dizziness or sweatiness. They are the bodily symptoms that represent how you feel.

Causes – Causes are the deeper roots of why you've fallen victim to burnout. Some examples are working conditions, grief, relationships, and trauma or money problems. They are the long-term cause of your burnout that needs to be addressed, preferably with people from your inner circle or professional helpers.

Solutions – Solutions are the things you can do to get out of your burnout. Again, the way into the burnout is often not the same as the way out. We should pay attention to the causes of burnout, but tackling emotional signals, triggers and symptoms can be just as helpful in making you stronger again.

Gathering Phase

Now you know why I find sharing my experience with you so important. I wish there had been someone out there who could have told me about the 'panic trick' much sooner. My anxiety disorder put lots of pressure on my relationship to the point we had to restart in a way that was better for us both. So I hope that by reading this book, you can avoid this kind of unnecessary added stress during your recovery.

The lesson here is that while you need to gather advice and experiment with it, you don't have to cling to it too quickly. It is understandable you are frantically looking for answers. Try taking a breather (preferably from the belly) and allow yourself some time to look for your personal solutions. Take one step back for two steps forward.

Besides, looking at all those aspects of burnout is actually interesting. It not only teaches us about ourselves but it also highlights in what kind of crazy society we sometimes find ourselves living. Letting all the aspects of burnout sink in will give you the clarity you crave. Plus, learning about all the solutions out there is very useful, even without burnout. They can all make your life better, regardless of your condition right now.

You will meet with some resistance in this gathering phase. People really want to help you, so they will tell you everything they know. Unfortunately, not all their advice will help you recover. I've lost count of how many people suggested taking a long vacation for instance, only to find out that when I did, things got worse. Burnout is inside of you, so you carry it with you wherever you go.

This doesn't mean you should drop your holiday plans! Again, it's all highly personal. So if you can skip town, by all means do it. I just wanted to point out that in the kindness of people's counsel, their solutions may not always work *for you*. Also, some people will be offended if you ignore their recommendations, even people very close to you. It's called 'projecting'; they assume what works for them will work for you too.

Trying to convince people that I needed to take my own path proved hard at times. Your professional helper will have a different opinion than your sibling, whose opinion will differ from that of your friend, who will say something different than your lover.

Again, just a couple of examples from my own experience. A friend and brilliant psychiatrist, who helped me greatly, once advised me to go to a psychologist. This psychologist told me he couldn't help me and advised mindfulness training for me.

To this day, people still don't get why going to a psychologist didn't work for me. It worked for them, so it *should have worked for me*. That's what many people think! Then my haptonomist – who was my biggest saving grace – didn't think mindfulness would work for me, but it did. She was right about almost everything... except that.

See what am I getting at? Even the absolute best helpers are not always right. So let me give you the one bit of advice that *is* guaranteed to work: don't ignore advice, but also don't assume it's the answer. If you take a broad approach, gather all the counsel you can, keep your expectations low and your mind open, experiment a little and then chose your own path, you will increase your chances of a quicker recovery.

Openly exploring your options is your first opportunity to regain control and will help make your journey less stressful.

Negative and Positive Emotions

The reason I might be able to help you as part of your Help Team is that, although I am not a burnout guru, I *am* both a writer and a musician. This means I am qualified to talk to you about something hugely important to your process: your emotions.

I am actually somewhat of an expert on emotions. Not only do I know what to do to evoke emotions through my music, speeches, interviews and books, I also studied emotions extensively when I wrote a book on emotional needs and wants of people, resulting in an emotional index that is used worldwide by many people today.

And because I am a creative person, I have frequently been exposed to the usual pitfalls such as feeling depressed when a work is finished or the infamous 'writer's block'. Even during my burnout – which was admittedly caused by emotional neglect – I never stopped delving into the subject of emotions. My research on it spans decades.

With my profession, comes a deeper understanding of all emotions, including the negative ones. You should be aware that lots of the feelings we will be covering are negative. Negative emotions are not fun. But it is crucial you learn to embrace and understand them. As signals, they are just as important as positive emotions.

Just so you know, most of my other creative work has a more positive and loving and encouraging tone. In this book however, I've taken a more balanced approach between positive and negative emotions. So occasionally, I'm going to be cynical or stoic or sad or angry. I do this because I know this reflects the emotions you are going through right now.

It is important for you to understand that I've been there and I will not sugar coat anything. Shying away from the negative will not help you get to the positive restart you so badly long for. I want to connect with you through the negative and turn that around, so we can come out seeing all of this burnout experience as a positive opportunity.

I'm also a Dutchman. As a rule, the Dutch can be very blunt. For the purposes of your recovery, I've fully embraced that attitude! My words will therefore occasionally be harsh, confrontational or surprising to you. But in the end, they will help you emerge reborn. Again, we need to focus on the painful, not avoid it. We'll look pain straight in the eyes... and discover it really isn't as bad as you might think right now.

The trick will be to focus on the 'right' pain, at the right moment. Although you might not immediately notice, I've carefully selected the order of the subjects we need to look at. This is not a set order, and you should feel free to pick and mix according to your needs. It's not so much a step-by-step plan either because, despite what many burnout professionals will tell you, with burnout there is no such thing as step-by-step guide.

Yet the sequence I've chosen does have a certain emotionally relevant order to it. I will present everything as clearly and concisely as possible. We won't rush through it, don't worry. Haste is not the same as speed. So, I will vary the speed in which I tell you things, simply because I know you'd like answers with a certain degree of tempo. So without further ado, let's begin with the most important lesson you need to learn.

Acceptance, Surrender and Letting Go

Since you're probably going through hell right now and are frantically looking for answers, let's open with the most important thing you will need to learn: surrender.

Here's the lowdown. The way out of your burnout is to accept that the signals your body and mind are giving to you, especially the uncomfortable ones, are completely and utterly natural. Fight these symptoms and they will not dissolve. Accept them – surrender to them and you can let them go, making way for your recovery.

Let these signals flow through you, however scary they are. You've got to stop swimming against the tide and accept that you have been hit by burnout. That may sound simple, but letting go is always hard, even without burnout. The very reason you have landed in this situation is because you were swimming against the current in the first place. You are used to the struggle and have been strong enough to keep it up for a long time.

Strangely enough, falling into a burnout is a sign of strength. It's strong people who get hit hardest by burnout because they can swim better than others. Problem is, you've been swimming in the wrong direction, for too long. Even the strongest can't do that forever.

To correct this and change direction, your subconscious mind has now protested in the form of a shock to your body, mind and soul. It knows that the direction you chose to swim in is no longer the right one. So it is giving you signals, including the ever-present 'couch potato' signal.

In other words, your subconscious is asking you to become that couch potato for a while to give it time to restructure. It is begging you to surrender to this process. If you refuse the couch, it will restructure anyway, but it will be a more forceful procedure. So go ahead, lay on the couch. You know you need the break...

... so take that break already!

Comfy? Then you're ready to hear this: a burnout is a reboot. Your system is correcting and rewiring itself, which is literally an unstoppable process. To add insult to injury, you have very little control over it. In a way, the tide has grown so powerful that you will have no other choice than to be dragged along with its current.

If you can accept that you no longer have control, things will become easier. And although it is an unstoppable process, it is possible to help that rewiring along, provided you are willing to change your state of mind. Just think of it like this: most of the time it is good to fight for things. But sometimes in life, the way to win is to surrender. This is one of those moments.

In other words: trust the tide.

That sounds terrible, but is in fact the opposite: it's an opportunity. You heard it right! Your couch is an opportunity. For those of us who are control freaks (aren't we all?), this 'letting go' will at first feel like mental torture. That feeling *will* pass. It will eventually be replaced by a eureka moment, although you probably don't believe that right now.

No matter - let's just continue with what you're physically experiencing right now... and why.

Part II: Waking the Animal

What is happening to you?

Pick your symptoms: pain, depression, chronic fatigue, insomnia, anxiety, paralyzing fear, dizziness, lack of sleep, strained relationships, confusion, detachment, vagueness, no sex drive, nausea, a lack of appetite, impaired concentration, anger, isolation, forgetfulness...

It all sucks.

These emotions? They are signals or signs similar to Defcon alerts. They could be related to your work, your relationship, your friends, your family (oh... always the family!), your past, your diet or your habits, your surroundings, your experiences or all of the above. We will go deeper into that later. Right now, let's focus on understanding what is happening *to* you and why. And let's drop that bomb right now.

Your cortisol levels are too high.

Cortisol is the so-called 'stress hormone'. It is not bad. But right now, your body is producing too much of it. That's not dangerous per se, but other hormones that make you naturally feel good, like dopamine, serotonin and endorphins, are not able to counter this increase effectively. They will in time, if you allow your body and mind rest.

Burnout is best described in racing terms when it refers to the moment a driver 'burns out' their tires with a show of smoke, a sort of 'overdrive', for the crowd's amusement. It's a good analogy. You have come into your burnout because your conscious mind has been pushing your body and soul into a state of spectacular overdrive.

To cope with this state of headlong overdrive – to keep up with all of the things happening in your life and your mind essentially - your body has been tricked into producing the chemicals and hormones it would normally produce in genuinely life-threatening situations. Your busy life with all of its pressures has become a simulated life threat within your body. It is not a *real* threat, but we'll discuss that in detail later.

The cortisol hormone is natural, useful and good. It teaches: your body produces it in circumstances when you need to adapt and learn new behaviour that will benefit your survival. That is why cortisol levels are usually highest when you wake up. The morning is the best moment to teach and experience beneficial behaviour to your health.

It is also produced by our bodies to fend off the common cold and is meant to warn us of stressful moments, spurring us into action. It is most commonly known as the 'fight, flight or freeze' hormone. It's a natural chemical that urges us to respond to danger. It is also produced to give you adrenaline when you need it. All in all it's an action-oriented hormone.

However, in response to prolonged exposure to stress, anxiety, sadness or other negative emotions, your body has gotten used to being in a sort of 'spectacular overdrive' and is overproducing cortisol, leaving you in a state of perpetual 'fight or flight' mode, or at least somewhere close to it.

In other words, your mind is tricking you into thinking that *everything* is now a dangerous situation and so you express classic signs of burnout, such as anxiety in the grocery store, crowds, social situations, confined spaces or at work... you name it. Your body is now seeing danger, sadness and negativity everywhere, even if it's not really there. It's on constant 'overdrive', and it's 'burning you out'.

How did this happen? And what should your first response be?

First Response

While solutions are very personal, there is one thing that all of us 'patients' have in common: anxiety and depression. That is why what I'm about to tell you is probably the most important thing you need to know right now: you'll have to learn to let these emotions flow through you and ride them out, preferably without trying to do anything about them (except maybe writing them down to calm yourself down).

In essence, the moment you get these feelings, recognize them for what they are: just feelings. Like a headache, you feel uncomfortable, but it will pass. Let those feelings do their thing for a while, and they will flow away again. Just acknowledge them and become aware of them. Tell yourself this: your thoughts are not facts. They are important signals, but not reality.

Let's demonstrate this by focusing on one of the more pronounced symptoms of burnout, the panic attack. Leading psychologist David Carbonell, who has written a book on the subject entitled *The Panic Attack Workbook,* talks about the 'panic trick'. This is the trick: just thinking of panic will spark a panic attack. The very thought of panic alone is enough.

Panic attacks make you feel terrible, so naturally you don't want them to occur. You develop countermeasures to keep them at bay, such as avoiding places and situations, developing protective rules, rituals, or superstitions. Or, you come to count on certain support people or chosen objects and distractions to keep you 'safe'. They may work for the time being, but when you come to rely on them, they will only serve as reminders of the panic, fuelling your panic further.

It's a nasty trick, but a trick nonetheless. Countermeasures don't work in the long run. Why? Because there never was a real threat to begin with! If you want to get rid of those panic attacks, you need to learn *not* to use countermeasures and simply let the feelings flow through you, however terrible they may be. After all, the feelings are not facts.

I highly recommend reading Carbonell's book if you suffer from panic attacks. For now however, I'd like to present Carbonell's perspective: Whatever you are feeling, you can let it flow through you. Observe and acknowledge the feelings instead of letting them take over. This goes for panic attacks, but also for all of the other symptoms we suffer during burnout.

Feeling tension, sadness or fatigue are things that everybody experiences. *They are normal.* We even go to scary or sad movies to experience them! But if you go to the movies, you have a choice of which emotions you want to experience. Right now, you are experiencing emotions without having that choice.

They are the same feelings you could have in a normal, non-burnout situation: feelings that can pass through you and dissolve. Plus, we have a lot of ways of expressing our emotions and making sense of them. We'll explore many of these a bit further on.

For now, if you are overwhelmed by panic at some point, call the emergency line to get yourself an ambulance! Trust me, the emergency personnel won't think you're foolish. They deal with anxiety patients everyday. And rather than something *really* detrimental happening to you, they would prefer to make sure you are ok. There should be no embarrassment about getting the help you need, whatsoever.

Just think of it like this: burnout is the world's number one affliction right now. Guess who are near the top of that list? Yes, medical professionals! Trust me, they know.

All right... is your immediate panic dropping? Then let's slow down a little. The way out of your burnout is more about a thousand tiny steps than it is about one big one. And it starts with an emotional step: letting go of pride.

Letting Go of Pride

Calling that ambulance is what millions of people have done. Calling your loved ones and crying your heart out is another thing that millions of us have done. You are anxious, depressed, tired... it is best if you listen to those signals and let them flow like the rivers they are right now. Share them in abundance.

And that brings us to the emotion of pride. Burnout is most common among people who have relatively successful lives. And almost everyone who has fallen victim to it, didn't think it would happen to them. Including me. I did know I was close to it, but I thought I could somehow dodge the burnout. That I was the exception. I was quite proud too.

But the truth is I hadn't developed the right tools yet to cope with stress. And if you have a successful career and family life and such, you can feel that it is not your place to have a burnout. You feel as if you shouldn't be complaining or making a fuss about it, or that within your 'circle of friends and co-workers' it will be seen as weakness. Worried about how it looks to others, you feel embarrassed - even ashamed.

But while you may wish otherwise, here's some tough love: sorry to bust your bubble but the burnout is here buddy.

The prouder you are about not giving in, admitting or accepting it, the more vulnerable you will become in the long run. As I mentioned before, it is often the strong-willed who fall victim to burnout. Which is exactly why I will use some strong, blunt words with you right now: forget about your image to the outside world. It is not important!

Now before you start feeling depressed about that too... this is actually a really, really good thing! According to

German burnout guru Markus Pawelzik, burnouts occur because of both external and internal expectations. So a good step is to let those expectations go for now.

Remember, you are rewiring from the inside. You are becoming more 'you', so you really don't have to think of how others will judge you. So how does this work? Let's look at the group of people who always have the highest expectations on everything: perfectionists.

Lowering expectations

Perfectionists put such high expectations on themselves because they feel they can achieve anything. The catch is that they start to experience stress every time they don't meet their own expectations.

This is not linked to a career per se. Many housewives or stay-at-home dads can put huge pressure on themselves to 'perform' in family and friend circles. Or feel they have 'failed' because they have trouble juggling their work and family lives.

It's all about how they feel based on their own expectations. In this example, once they would accept that literally *everyone* has trouble balancing work and family, their expectations lower together with their stress levels.

So this is a trigger or a cause of burnout that comes from the inside: what it is we feel based on what we expect in our own minds. But stress can also arise because of external factors: the impossible expectations of a boss, a loved one, family members, a particular environment, event or a social circle.

This kind of external pressure – especially when experienced over a prolonged time period - can leave you feeling incompetent and insecure while in reality, the problem is not you. It's them.

My point is that if you want those internal or external expectations to get to a more realistic level the first emotion you will have to leave behind is pride. The irony of course, is that pride is a dominant emotion in successful people who value their reputations. This makes it especially tough to shake.

But it's now about you, and not about others. Pride really is the most damaging emotion to your recovery. It undercuts all the efforts and keeps throwing you back to square one. So you can and must shake it.

Yet letting go of pride is just a first step. You will learn that if you let go of pride, you open the door to another emotion that can be equally stressful in its own right: feeling vulnerable.

On Emotional Signals

During a burnout, feeling vulnerable is terrifying, but you do get used to it. In time you can even learn to use that feeling to your advantage. The trick will be to recognize when vulnerability is giving you a false or an accurate signal. Example: if you feel vulnerable skydiving, it's accurate. But feeling vulnerable while waiting in line at the supermarket?

Emotions are physiological signals from the mind, encouraging us to react to a situation. They are often involuntary gut reactions, which we can control a second or so later. These signals originate in the oldest parts of our brain - where they form instantly – and then they flow into the newer parts of our brain, giving us a chance to figure out a logical response.

In some cases, the emotional signal will not reach the newer, more rational part of our brain, simply because the context is too overwhelming. Another example: if a big grizzly bear would walk into your room right now, you don't have the chance to overanalyze the situation. Instead, your emotions kick in and your so-called 'lizard' brain takes over, forcing you to respond on the spot with a fight, flight or freeze response.

Sorry I've dialled the anxiety level up a bit, but I'm trying to prove a point. Go ahead, look around for the grizzly in the room... I know you want to. Feeling safe? Then let's move on!

Actually, this imaginary situation is exactly what we want to talk about. Most likely you have felt a tiny little alarm go off in your mind when you thought of that bear. This is because the more rational part of your mind – which has developed later in the evolutionary process of mankind – is able to imagine things that may not even be real. This ability, what in ancient Greece was known as 'logos' (logic), is what sets us apart from animals.

We can imagine stories, films, music and more great stuff like that! This imagination is what makes us human.

But we can also imagine having a heart attack while standing in line at the supermarket, a grizzly bear in our room, or a terrorist in the crowd. You can also imagine how an ex feels about you, what your boss, commander or friends might think of you knowing you are in a burnout. Or you take it further and imagine what would happen to you if you lost your job or got divorced.

And here's the kicker; *even if none of this is really happening, you can still feel it*. We can imagine things in the new part of our brain... and then communicate it to the old. Thoughts are not facts. But we can sure as hell still *feel* them.

In a normal situation, you'd be able to dismiss those thoughts as not being real. In a burnout-cortisol-spectacular-overdrive situation, fear and vulnerability are heightened in your mind and then translated into a physiological reaction of the body: fight, flight or freeze. Your adrenaline levels go up and so does your blood pressure.

(Fun fact for those who feel they are going to faint in such a situation: you probably won't. In order to faint, your blood pressure must drop instead of go up! If you do faint, you might want to talk to your doctor for medication to counter low blood pressure.)

What we need to do in general is get those cortisol levels down. The 'how' will be more fully presented in the Solutions chapter. For now, it is important to understand that those negative emotions are caused by a failure to recognize when your vulnerability is real and when it is simulated in your mind.

Waking the Animal

Paradoxically, if there were a real threat to your life, you would probably not be that anxious at all! Instead, you'd automatically switch to lizard brain autopilot. I've experienced such a situation even. It was during a full-blown-anxiety-over-the-top period when I was driving and found myself in a life-threatening situation on the road.

I just responded with my gut. It was the right response. I felt no fear, no anxiety whatsoever. So the best way to recognize the distinction between a real or imagined threat is to get emotional, to tap *into* that lizard brain. We need to wake your inner animal. As a matter of fact, the very reason the modern world's number one affliction is now burnout, is because so many of us ignore this emotional animal within.

We over-think and under-feel.

As a writer and musician, I'm frequently asked to give lectures on how to spark creativity within organisations. I always start those lectures with the same question: who in the room has ever fallen in love? This gets the same response every time. From the get go, everybody gets nervous and starts to laugh. Everyone in the crowd raises their hands. Yes, they know love... thank God.

Then I ask them to describe the feeling if 'the person you are in love with were to enter the room right now'. This is the moment when confusion sets in. They describe how they get nervous, sweaty, turn red and want to laugh and kiss and hug, and how it's the greatest feeling in the world.

But there is always at least one person who points out that the feeling can also be *absolutely terrifying*. That's because being in love also means you will lose all control of your rational mind. Literally.

Studies show that when you're in love, there is no activity left in the newer part of your brain - absolutely none. You have no choice but to give in to the feeling, to the animal - no matter the outcome.

You. Are. Vulnerable.

That's the moment when I have the crowd exactly where I want them: deeply panicked. To hammer it in, I ask them to describe what would happen in our previous example: a grizzly bear has just walked into the room. How do you feel now? They then start to describe emotions that are eerily similar to the dread of being in love: no control.

The crowd expects me to teach them what methods they can use to become more creative, but there are none. All creative processes are about letting go. Instead I teach them they are *already* creative.

Creativity is a survival instinct. Deep in our DNA are the genes that spark creativity as a method for resolving any situation – from danger to love - in a split second. This also includes being highly creative, as when singing or writing poetry.

Everyone has the creative gene. I just remind the crowd to let their gut take over. I don't teach them, I get them to feel. Which is precisely what I'm hoping you will do too. I want you to *feel,* not *think.*

But there is a catch. Releasing the animal inside of you is basically the opposite of what we do in our modern living and working environments. It will spark friction in your daily life.

In a way we need to teach our rational minds that we don't always have to be so damned rational about everything. However, this has become increasingly difficult in a society that is filled to the brim with burnout triggers.

It has become so pervasive that I can actually make money by teaching people how to reconnect with their inner animal. This brings us to our first major trigger of burnouts: modern society.

Modern Society

Most of us no longer face immediate threats to our lives in today's world. We don't have to hunt for food or deal with grizzly bears anymore. In theory, anxiety levels should be going down drastically. So why are they going up? Why has burnout become an epidemic?

We spend a lot of our time on computers and mobile phones, chasing deadlines, running to appointments or meetings and have full agendas. Bright lights surround us in our sterile offices. We have TV's, cars, airplanes, sirens, traffic lights, cigarettes, alcohol, rent or mortgages, drugs – prescription or not - fatty food, and incredibly realistic computer games.

We have the news. Natural disasters, dictators and terrorists reach our lives everyday. We are supposed to take responsibility for our energy consumption, plus use healthy and environmentally friendly products to counter global warming. And on top of all that, we cope with a daily barrage of advertisements constantly trying to activate our consumer instincts.

Then there's social media, movies and TV telling us how great our life would be if we had a happy home life, wealth, a great career, an amazing body by working out like crazy, a superb dating life, wife or husband, the company of our friends, and enjoyed the latest trends... just for starters. All the while drinking cup after cup of coffee.

There is a reason why people who actually *do* live in areas with grizzly bears *don't* get burnouts! They live in a natural environment that more closely resembles the world in which our species evolved.

From an instinctive, animal point of view, they are home. For them, the difference between real and simulated danger is clear. For us...it's less so.

In the modern world our bodies and minds are constantly dealing with all kinds of situations that generate at least some level of stress. At the same time our tolerances for stress have been reduced because we spend very little time just *being*. Instead we feel we must do things all the time and use our time efficiently and effectively.

We forget that downtime – the art of doing nothing – is extremely important for our bodies and minds to relax and reset.

And with our modern media we create the illusion that we are able to control all aspects of life. So when life does throw us a curveball, we don't know how to react to it. I'd even argue that newer generations – including my own generation and me personally - are actually *less* capable of dealing with life's hardships than the generations before them.

Just think of it: we burn out from modern life. While people who survived the Second World War don't even know what that last sentence even *means*.

About your senses

Now, I'm not saying that our modern living conditions alone have directly caused your burnout. In fact, I'd bet they haven't unless you are extremely sensitive to triggers. Plus, many of you readers are here because of deeper and more serious causes.

Still, we really do need to talk about those modern day circumstances. They may not be the cause of a burnout. But they function as a constant distraction and are quite possibly the triggers that are part of a burnout. That's because they tend to desensitize you to the reality of your 'inner' emotional grizzly.

I mean 'desensitize' very literally. When you suffer from burnout you are not fully connected to your senses. You are stuck in a stressful thinking pattern, meaning you have a hard time connecting to the world around you. Your senses are either too sensitive or not sensitive enough. Let's give some examples.

Sometimes you are unable to hear what people are saying because you have drifted off too far. Or the opposite; you become very sensitive to sound in general, making it hard to cope with the noises around you. This also happens to the other senses sight, touch, smell and taste. In a burnout situation they can all be affected in some way. In time they will return to normal of course. For now, at least you are aware of this.

Modern society also creates expectations, many of which are impossible to fulfil. All those expectations and ambitions can be fine when you're feeling good and know where you are going. However the moment things aren't going well in your life, you can be confronted with the fact that your senses are on full alert all the time.

But the alarm bells you're hearing are drowning out the alerts you *should* be paying attention to: your gut.

To illustrate this, let's talk about a persistent myth that is an example of how we think about our modern lives: the idea that children can cope with technology better than adults. To a degree, this can be true. If you learn something at a young age, it becomes second nature.

But as I argued before, it could also mean the opposite: children are *less* able to cope with life because of technology. The physiology of children is still the same as that of past generations. Technology hasn't suddenly and magically become part of our biology. Yet we now use it more than ever.

As a result, we are seeing young children on prescription drugs, an increase in kids with autistic challenges (closely linked to trigger sensitivity) and young adults suffering from an identity crisis.

Nowadays, burnout is especially common for those between the ages of 20 and 30. In other words: all evidence points to a massive and widespread sensory overload.

That's very, very alarming. The persistence of this myth - that says children can better cope with technology than adults - reveals just how desensitized we have become to our true human emotional nature.

We even flat out deny it in our kids.

The Pursuit of Happiness

So let's consider 'how' kids are happy. Did you know that the happiest children on Earth are the Dutch? According to children's organisation Unicef, Dutch kids hold the number one happiness spot. The most important reason is attributed to the fact that children in the Netherlands are allowed to roam unsupervised by their parents and teachers.

They bike to school by themselves, without helmets. They don't have to learn math, reading and writing until they express the wish to do so. They don't compete in class. They play outside in schoolyards and parks without their parents looming over them. To a degree, they are even left to experiment with alcohol and marihuana during adolescence.

For many of my non-Dutch readers, this sounds scary as hell. How can you leave your children so unsupervised? How can you not encourage your kids to compete at a young age? How can you let them come into contact with drugs? In some countries you would face an army of lawyers suing you over such liberal practices. Yet in the Netherlands, it has proven to work. Overwhelmingly.

Essentially kids are taught that they can be kids. When they fall from the bike and hit their head, it is considered a good thing. They learn to get back up again, that life doesn't always give you a safety helmet and that they should be more careful the next time.

By giving them freedom, they learn that 'shit happens' and they automatically teach *themselves* responsibility.

So despite outside appearances, the Dutch grow up to be more conservative than you'd think. It's a paradox: by giving so much freedom, the kids learn at a young age how to take care of themselves and more importantly… what not to do.

So you get entire generations that have a lot more control over their lives later on. It's ultimately about confidence. Kids don't grow up in fear of what *could* go wrong. They stay in the moment and learn what you should do *when* something does go wrong.

How different this is for a grown-up, including for this Dutch one. Our Western societies are geared to always strive for something in the future. That happiness is always on the horizon and not in the now.

For Dutch kids, all emotions are in the now. Including happiness. It's not something that more money, a new wardrobe or a flashy career gives you. It's just a feeling, nothing more. Happiness is not something you strive for in the future, *it's a state of being in the now*.

You can't pursue happiness. If you try to do that, you get depressed because it is not something you can 'catch'. Happiness is already inside of you. You can evoke it anytime you feel like it.

You don't *get* happy, you *are* happy.

Yet our entire society seems to encourage the pursuit of 'getting more'. Ambition and innovation are the keywords of our day. And although it is commendable to strive for better things in the future, it is also stressful.

It means that we always feel a little depressed about not having those things that are waiting on the horizon. And when we do reach that horizon, we are disappointed because it didn't meet our high expectations.

Our minds are literally pushed out of the real world moment and into a fictitious ideal. And when we don't succeed in achieving that fiction, our minds dwell on the past as we contemplate our perceived 'failures'. And then the cortisol increases.

The Cortisol Rises

In modern society, the availability of positive experiences is far more abundant as compared to the past. This leads to a situation in which we are continuously invited to have greater expectations for our future. Experiencing positive emotions has an effect on our brain, adding serotonin, dopamine and endorphins. In short, we feel good.

These hormones are addictive. Our minds and bodies are geared towards experiencing them again and again. We push ourselves to go after more, taking us further beyond the now. An even better presentation, an even greater audience, even more money or more likes on social media. We become addicted to this confirmation that keeps us wanting what we don't yet have.

Simply put: our lives are so full of possibilities, we tend to put too much on our plates. We end up trying to do everything at once: a successful career, lots of sports, entrepreneurship, parenthood, going out with friends, increasingly spectacular holidays, while multitasking our way through binge watching whatever grabs us.

All the while, the hundreds of media messages we receive everyday are telling us of the great life we can have, fuelling our hopes, dreams and most importantly, our expectations. In a way, we are emotionally spoiled. Even if we cannot obtain a certain status, we live in a world that is constantly telling us that we can if we just try harder.

If you truly experience constant joy doing all of this, you probably aren't reading this book! For the rest of us however, a subtle change starts to occur. We are subconsciously starting to feel as if all of these things are an obligation instead of a joyful experience. Deep inside we start to feel we *need* six-pack abs, *need* a great career, *need* to watch this show, *need* to have a family, *need to need...*

The Power of the Mind

There is a tipping point between what we *want* and what we *need.* When you reach this tipping point, your body start to produce more cortisol so you can take action to meet your *needs.*

In essence, we tell our bodies that our joyful *wants* have become our *needs to survive.* Such is the power of our minds that now all of a sudden missing out on something fun is experienced by our body as a life-threatening situation. Enter the cortisol.

Over time, this build-up of cortisol will backfire. Your body and mind will start to resist those things you thought you 'needed'. Your body now labels these simulated 'needs' as 'bad'. It becomes a vicious cycle. The result: your body presses the pause button.

Of course, striving for things on the horizon is not a bad thing. But we have rationalized it as an endless pursuit. We have pushed our feelings of happiness into the future instead of keeping them in the now. We keep adding to the tension of our suspended happiness and fail to experience *joie de vivre* in the moment.

Enjoying an ice cream cone in the now doesn't even occur to us anymore. Sure, we are eating it, but while we take a bite we're thinking of something else instead of savoring the ice cream as a child would.

And when that fantastic band starts to play, we grab our mobile phones to tape it for future use or share it with everyone. We don't even think about just closing our eyes anymore and letting the music flow over us...

It's a shame. And it's hurting us. We have become disconnected from our emotions in the now. And there's only one way left to reconnect - waking up our inner animal!

Drowning out the noise

To wake up the animal inside, we have to completely turn off to what society throws at us for a while. Say no to the things that don't suit you. Say no to people, to media, to bad influences... no and no! A great way to quickly reduce your stress, anxiety and depression levels is to step back and take a break from modern life, and realign with what is truly important to you: feeling happy.

So get rid of a few triggers first. Taking this step will help you build a solid base for recovery because it will make you directly reconnect with your more basic and personal instincts. In other words, it will drown out the noise.

So what am I talking about? Well, turn off your TV to start with. Try not to spend too much time on the Internet or any screen. Cut porn. Social media is one of the biggest triggers of stress too (the 'fear of missing out'), so I recommend disconnecting for a while. Really, just log out. You'll thank me for that later.

The news is also a trigger I recommend avoiding. News is almost always negative. And when you're suffering from burnout, it helps if you don't have to think about all the bad people out there. But even more important, the news is *out of your control*.

If we want to drown out the noise, we can start by letting go of those things we can't control. You can't control what an ex puts on Facebook, or what a crazy person or even the president might do. And every time you do tune into those things, you will be left with a sense of hopelessness for not being able to do anything. So, skip it all together. Tune into yourself and tune out what you can't control.

So what *can* you do? Get into nature. Read a good book. Play squash. Go out and take photos... that kind of stuff. It may sound like skimpy advice, but such things literally put your brain into a much more natural state - in the here and now. And that is the most important thing your burned-out-self needs to do right now.

Such simple small steps allow you to listen to internal *signals* instead of the external *noise*. I know it's not easy to disconnect from all the noise in the world. That's ok. You can take it slow. It's hard to face your negative emotions, especially your fears. But every time you do, you will feel better afterwards... and probably stronger.

You also don't have to do it all in one go. So forgive yourself if you binge-watched that show (I did!) or if you checked your email or tuned in to catch the latest news. It's ok - really it is. Forgive yourself.

Just try not to close down emotionally by seeking out only the noise around you. I know it sounds terrible, digging into your emotions. But once I disconnected, I personally started to rather enjoy it as a sort of 'deprivation' that brought me closer to my real self.

I learned to trust again in what my gut had to tell me, even if it was anger or sadness or fear. I felt honestly alive again, and so will you. Cutting out the 'noise' and getting back to yourself can even change your posture; shifting your energy from high in your shoulders and neck to all the way down and low in your belly where it's supposed to be: in your groin.

Let go of control. You may even lose control a little when we dive into the causes of your burnout. You have your Help Team at the ready if it becomes a little too much to bear. Trust me, it'll be nice to have that sense of basic instinct back in your life. It will mean you are finally ready to look at the causes of your burnout.

Trust that instinct... you animal.

Part III: Causes of Burnout

Working Environments

Ok… inner animal: check. Now we can begin to focus on causes. Let's start with work. How does that feel for you?

Working environments can be very stressful, especially if they involve high expectations. The pressure of performing can be so great at times that it leaves you feeling you can never do enough. The perfectionists among you will recognize this instantly. But you don't have to be a perfectionist to crumble under job pressure. It happens to the best of us and to some degree, *all* of us.

Generally speaking, work stress is not a bad thing. Ambition has advanced the human race and your personal ambitions can lead you to great accomplishments. If however the pressure is put on you for an extensive period of time, while at the same time you don't feel confident that you can manage it, the cracks will start to show.

So back away from work… even if this means you are in danger of losing your job. I'm going to be very direct with you here and only say this once: no job is worth keeping if it causes you burnout. It's one of the most common stories surrounding the phenomenon: "*I burned out at work, quit my job and now I'm happy*".

But there is more. Even when there is no pressure at all, work can *still* be stressful. This has to do with the physical aspects of many modern day workplaces: our offices and technology. Working environments tend to be very unnatural and can cut you off from your natural instincts.

The strong lights, the extensive amount of coffee (a huge anxiety trigger), greasy lunches, the stress of the commute and long meetings can combine to make you a stranger to yourself before you've even noticed.

Especially working on a computer for an extended time can increase stress levels, even if the job itself is not in the least bit stressful! It's a physical thing. When you are sitting still, your blood flow decreases. But doing mental work means your brain needs the blood upstairs. To cope, your body resorts to all kinds of tricks, including increasing cortisol to make up the difference.

This example is a perfect reminder of why I'm writing this book. Yes, many burnouts are caused by deep emotional problems! But sometimes all that stress can be caused by something more mundane... like sitting still for hours at a time, for days, weeks or even years without getting enough exercise. This cause of burnout is purely physical.

Just like working in construction can put you at risk of becoming physically injured, today's knowledge workers can become mentally injured. Afflictions suffered in your climate controlled office are different of course, but they are serious injuries – requiring treatment - just the same.

And even if your burnout has a deeper emotional cause, this can be amplified by a general lack of exercise. Some of you are in this burnout situation because of very deep emotional reasons, and I don't want to be disrespectful of their importance. But I'm also writing this book for those of you who may need a change of lifestyle rather than deep-diving into your soul.

Of course, changing your lifestyle can be equally hard as diving into the depths of your feelings. Remember that for each of us, burnout is highly personal. And although the reasons may be different, the symptoms all of you are experiencing are still very similar.

Emotions and Countermeasures

Stress at work can have multiple causes. Sometimes it has to do with the high expectations that your boss, your colleagues (external) or you yourself (internal) are putting on you. But even in a situation where the expectations are not that high, the physical factors can play a big part - and even be the very cause - of your burnout.

Whatever the cause of stress at work, there is something important you should know about its effect: emotions have a tendency to be contagious. We are social animals after all, who pick up each other's vibes.

So the stress that individuals experience can spread to everyone in the office, accumulating into more stress than is actually needed to do the work that needs to be done. It can even spread to society at large, which could explain at least part of the recent tensions in the world.

Your working environment can become a place where everyone is in constant survival mode – cortisol almost literally flying through the air - simply because people tend to mimic each other's emotions. Maybe the job that you and your colleagues are doing is not really that hard. But you *feel* it is impossible because of the simulated stress defining your environment.

I say 'simulated' because there is no actual danger in your office. But of course, what you feel is still very real. Thoughts are not facts, but you can feel them just the same. Long meetings, working hours, deadlines, and targets that are unrealistic can all add to this feeling.

Expectations… if they were suddenly gone, the actual job might not be so hard.

I'm pointing this out for a good reason: if you become conscious or mindful of your working environment and what it does to you, you will be able to develop countermeasures. Of course when work really is the core problem, you should walk away. But for some of you, this exercise in mindfulness might put things in perspective and make it possible for you to keep your job.

With this change in perspective, focusing on yourself in the 'here and now' versus letting your job always be geared towards a future result, gives you a choice. You can define and achieve future results by getting very stressed and pushing a lot of cortisol into your body to get going. Or you could choose to work on that future result by staying in the moment, feeling relaxed about what you're doing and enjoying the fact you are working to reach your goal, bettering yourself and your organisation.

It's all in *your* mind.

Your mind is powerful. This means it can focus on the negative with a lot of power. But it also means it can focus on the positive with exactly the same intensity.

Be mindful and you can develop your own tools to cope with stress. It can be as simple as taking regular breaks or getting some fresh air. Or, maybe listen to some reggae music next time you're in a train surrounded by less than relaxed commuters. In a flash, a stressful situation can turn into an inspirational one!

In fact, this mindfulness approach can help you cope with *all* busy or stressful situations, from traffic jams to pushy crowds at concerts... you name it.

So let's explore some possible feelings. Some of you already know you just have to quit. Some of you might feel your work really fits you, just not the organisation. Others might feel the type of work isn't suitable in the first place, or you might simply feel incompetent about doing it.

This however might just be a 'feeling' that signals you have low self esteem, while in reality you are very good at your job (and should feel high self esteem)! Or it might be a signal you need to stop being such a perfectionist or that the working environment needs to change... or your feelings towards it.

In any case, ask yourself the question: how does my job *feel*? And why? And get ready to be surprised.

Money Trouble

Work is of course also about making a living. Money problems are another common trigger or cause of burnout. Numerous studies have shown that people facing debt turn to their lizard brains, that older part of our mind that puts us in 'survival mode'. This survival mode makes it difficult for us to plan ahead or see the bigger picture, thus making it harder to solve problems.

Essentially our minds switch to short-term emotional thinking and have difficulty switching back to more rational long-term decision making. This means pressing the pause button here is also very difficult. You can lie on that couch. But that won't stop the bills from piling up.

It may sound strange, but I actually recommend embracing the survival mode in this case, at least for the time being. It puts you firmly into the moment. Setting yourself on 'survival' means you will make the hard decisions that help you deal with your immediate debt worries, releasing you from a huge amount of anxiety instantly. As long as you recognize that you are in lizard brain mode, you can make this work to your advantage.

When in debt, a little animal instinct goes a long way.

But there is one 'rational' decision that could help you immensely: let appropriate institutions or someone from your Help Team look into your finances. People who experience prolonged money problems have a tendency to hide them from the outside world, often unwittingly feeling embarrassed that they can't solve them themselves.

I was one of those people, as were many of my closest friends when they suffered money related stress. We each exhibited the same behaviour: we didn't talk about it. And even when the trouble became so overwhelming that we had to talk to someone about it, we still left things out.

We did not tell the whole story even when we were drowning in our bills.

Money is one of the most emotional subjects there is. We rationalize the pursuit of money in our society. Stock markets, loans, mortgages, credit cards, banks, insurance... they all have the appearance of being rational and controlled. This makes us think that we are failing at something that should be simple, as a rational and routine part of life.

Nothing could be further from the truth, as every stock market crash has proven... every time. Anything to do with money is complex and by definition very emotional.

Why? Because we need money to survive and unless society functions as a completely shared economy, this will continue to be the case. This explains all those studies that show we go into survival mode when we have money problems: we actually need to. We cannot escape the survival mode because if we do, we decrease our chances of survival!

It really doesn't get any more emotional. Speaking from experience, my advice here is to just acknowledge it. It is really quite common to have money issues. Just try not to fall into the trap that my friends and I did - thinking you are alone. It is perfectly normal to experience money stress in today's society. Reach out and you will see that you are not alone.

Your Relationships
So whom do we reach out to when we are in trouble?

Another common cause of burnouts is relationships whether romantic, family or friend oriented. If you identify this as a possible cause, your next step will feel terrible at first, but it will give you a great sense of relief later on: tell the people you have a strained relationship with that you need some distance, a pause or a break from your relationship with them.

Be prepared - this will most likely trigger a defensive response. If a person is the cause of your anxiety, than this person wants something from you that you cannot give at this moment in time. They are at odds with you. This means you *must* press pause with them or *you* will suffer the consequences, not them. And when you do press pause, they will no doubt feel offended in some way.

Brace yourself for only two possible outcomes to this situation. Either a person takes what you've told them into consideration, or the distance will grow bigger. Either way, you will be freed of the anxiety. I myself had to do this. It was painful at first, but it later restored those relationships. A little space can get you a lot of love in return.

Just think of it like this: the relationship is already damaged. Creating space is actually the thing that *heals* the relationship instead of damaging it further. So you are actually taking the step that helps to put things right. Distance gives us all time and space to heal.

I've had the pause button pushed *on* me as well: it was too hard for one of my loved ones to always deal with my burnout. Accepting this was hard, of course. You want people to help you, especially those who love you. But sometimes – due to whatever circumstances – they are not capable of doing that.

Even if it makes you very, very anxious at first, you must honour their feelings. And when you do, you will find it actually helps you because you are confronted with your emotions even more. It's painful, but it will help you heal and restore those relationships.

The fact that some people gave me space and I had to give space to others triggered me to heal faster. It showed me just how destructive a burnout could be to me and to others, and encouraged me to seek even more guidance. It pushed me to let go of the last shreds of pride and forced me to go over the threshold that healed me. Exactly what I needed.

I don't really have much else to tell you here, except to not censure your emotions. Some people may not be able to help you or even be the cause of your burnout.

Relationships may end, change, restore or become even better over time. It's a natural thing. It happens. Please don't blame others and don't blame yourself when distance is required. It's just one of those things you need to accept. It's a space you need to give to yourself.

Plus, there are always other options as you sort through your emotions and relationships. There are help lines you can call, online programs you can sign up for, professionals who can help and maybe other loved ones who can step up to the plate.

Remember you are never alone! There are millions of us and we all can recover! And when you recover, you will find that healing yourself will have a positive impact on your relationships with everyone else.

Trauma, Loss, Depression and Escape

Of course, sometimes we are not in a position to control relationships. When we experience loss, near loss, a breakup or a trauma that we could not prevent, this can add to our stress levels significantly. These situations are periods of grief even when they don't appear to be that at first glance.

Again I can teach you something from personal experience. One of the people closest to me had to undergo life-threatening surgery twice. It went well, thank goodness. But I later realized that, even though everything had turned out well, this emotional period was one of the main causes of my burnout. I had not dealt with my emotions surrounding the surgery, which directly added to the mountain of stress I was already under.

Of course, I ended up drinking and smoking. Others escape their feelings by binge watching or reaching for drugs. Still others dive into their work to escape or start obsessive training regimes to maintain a sense of control over their bodies.

None of the above is necessarily a bad thing. When we feel good about ourselves, a beer doesn't hurt. Diving into your work can be a really good thing. Exercise is something I would recommend to everyone. And binge watching is a lot of fun.

But when you are feeling down, all of these things tend to add to your problems.

Alcohol, nicotine, drugs, too much training, too much work or sitting in front of the TV all day... build up your cortisol levels even higher. From a physical standpoint, you are asking your body to cope with something while it is already in stress mode. From a mental point of view, you are escaping the emotions you need to face in order to recover.

While similar to burnout and sharing many of the same symptoms, I don't feel that grieving is the same as burnout. A symptom of grieving could be feeling lethargic. But the reason for your lack of energy is very different from the energy drain that burnout causes.

This is also true for 'classic' clinical depression: people who can't seem to enjoy the good things in life are not 'burned out' per se. And yes, similar observations can be made about Post Traumatic Stress Syndrome.

However there are similarities. I can again point out that the way *in*to a bad mental state – whether it is burnout, grief, trauma or clinical depression, might not be the same as getting *out*. The way out of your grief or depression could be similar to burnout solutions. In any of these cases, it is all about letting the emotions flow through you, accepting them and letting them go.

I should also briefly mention our disposition to negative emotions because it can explain a lot about causes. Some of us are naturally inclined to experience certain emotions in a way that other people wouldn't. I myself am a bit of a paradox in that sense. I have a natural tendency to strive for change. But when big changes do occur I also have a natural disposition to become anxious, even if I was the one instigating them.

I realize we are becoming ever more serious in this part of the book. We are discussing the deeper causes of your burnout and making necessary sidesteps into grief, depression, trauma and disposition, which isn't easy.

I want to inspire you to embrace and accept those negative emotions by reminding you that I had them too and they can be overcome. I'll slow the tempo down a bit so we can start floating towards the positive.

Floating Towards the Positive

When we discuss the causes of our burnouts, I want you to feel that it's ok to be sad, anxious and angry about things. As I said at the beginning of this book, I sometimes missed people simply acknowledging and connecting with the negative emotions I was experiencing, and nothing more.

So let's do that now.

Depression slows us down. We feel frustrated because we can't control the fact that it is there. However, we *can* change the way we *feel* about it. We can learn to see it as something positive, even looking at these emotional signals as opportunities to face our difficulties, learn to know ourselves better and make room for healing.

Giving space to what we feel is good even when it confronts us with the fact that we haven't been feeling good. So instead of pushing blindly ahead, maybe we can let these feelings trickle in. All we have to do now is acknowledge the emotions that are there. We don't have to immediately solve them. We can just let them be there for a while.

So now those emotions flow through you. Maybe you feel like crying, feel anger swelling up, or increased anxiety. Again, just let it be. Put down the book, close your eyes and let the emotions float around you.

And yes, if there is someone from your Help Team you can call and share those feelings with, go do it.

And when you've picked up these words again, maybe you will start to get some perspective. The perspective that your feelings are natural. The perspective that you are not alone. The perspective that your hormones need some TLC, or that relationships change.

Work is not always ideal. Money is always a tricky thing. And, sometimes you will get into situations you can't control. It sucks. But it's all part of life.

Just don't forget the perspective that things can change for the better. And that what is happening to you might be less of a disaster than you think. Remember that there are still opportunities out there, and that your recovery can happen as it has with millions of others.

You are rewiring your mind, and however painful, that's also an opportunity in your journey towards recovery.

There is hope.

And then, I hope you will sigh, and take a deep breath from your belly. Connect with your gut and drop your shoulders because those shoulders don't have to carry the world all alone.

When you do gain perspective you don't have to act immediately. Just let your inner animal take over, and know what you feel, without all the noise. This makes it possible for the other part of your brain - the logical part - to start to assemble solutions. In baby steps.

You have created space for your recovery.

Part IV:
Solutions

External and Internal Recognition

Remember that while tackling the causes of your burnout may be enlightening, it's not the only thing that can help you find your way out of burnout. Sometimes causes are just what they are. They need to be recognized but remain out of our control.

What you can control however is making use of a huge number of solutions that can help restore your confidence. So, still bearing in mind your path is personal, it's now time to look at the ones I have found for you.

Some of the solutions on these pages are geared towards internal issues, such as going to a psychologist or starting a meditation regime. Some of them offer ways of getting your hormone balance in order, and are more physical. Some of the solutions are presented to help you drown out the daily external noise that can overwhelm us. And I've added a lot of solutions you rarely hear about that actually work like a charm.

Each of these solutions is likely to help you in some way. They range from physical to emotional and from mental to spiritual. There is no particular order in which they are presented, but there is a certain emotional logic unique to each of them.

I'd like to again state that none of the solutions suggested are written in stone. The goal of this book is to give you perspective and options. Options that I will try to describe as best I can through my personal experience. Remember, I'm only part of your Help Team, and in the end only you can determine which solutions are best for you.

So feel free to pick and mix and experiment. And if you can, maybe have a little bit of fun. Instead of just letting the rewiring happen, you can now take an active role in directing it.

(Plus, if you feel like sharing your personal solutions with others, please let us know at www.restart-burnout-book.com!)

All I ask is for you to keep an open mind and to sometimes consider the unconventional. I encourage you to try things out, especially those things that initially seem strange to you. I too had to try things out that I thought were weird, only to learn that they actually helped me more than any medication would have.

Drum roll please…

Solution: Psychology

It should not come as a surprise that the first solution we are discussing is professional help. Don't be too proud to do this.

Seeking professional help is a sign of strength, not weakness. Facing your troubles means you've overcome your fear of them. It makes you a hero, because you are choosing to face them when you're most vulnerable. That takes *cojones*. Plus, psychologists are trained to deal with burnout and vulnerability anyway.

The best way to go about this is to shop around. Talking to a psychologist requires a certain 'click' between the two of you. You need to have the feeling they will understand you. So don't be afraid to do a few intake meetings before deciding on your psychologist. If they are any good, they will actually encourage that. And if they are really good, they will also tell you when they can help you or not.

Psychology is a broad field so there are many 'flavours' out there. Try to find yours and choose with your gut.

Solution: Haptotherapy

The second solution we can look at is a relatively new field developed in the 20th century in the Netherlands. It's called *haptonomy* or *haptotherapy* and is essentially a more holistic form of psychology that includes your physical body in the treatment. It teaches you to connect with your body, your surroundings and other people more easily.

The practice is a combination of talking about your emotions and then doing something physical in response to your feelings. For instance: hitting a punching bag if you've just discussed your inner anger or holding yourself if you've been feeling alone. And yes, I did both.

The philosophy behind it is that if you have mental injuries, they also manifest themselves in your body. Your emotions – which have an effect on your body - are the main focus.

The practice of haptonomy acknowledges the immense power of the emotional mind and how it affects your body directly. A simple example: if you feel down, your shoulders slump. If you feel stressed, your shoulders tighten. If you feel happy, your shoulders relax.

This differs from most psychological approaches that are about getting your head straight first. Haptotherapy doesn't just look at your mind but also at your emotions and your physical expression of them.

For me, this worked wonders. It quickly became my go-to therapy. My general practitioner recommended this over a psychologist. It was a personal choice that worked because of the physical aspects that urge you to express your emotions not just by talking, but also with physical games and movements.

It gave real world expression to what I felt inside, which was as exciting as it was uplifting.

Solution: Cognitive Behavioural Therapy

One of the more refined 'flavours' on the psychology menu is something called *Cognitive Behavioural Therapy*. This is a therapy focussed on slowly confronting your fears.

For instance, if you have a fear of heights, you will slowly be eased into situations involving your fear of heights and then gradually increase the interval and 'severity' of that confrontation. You face that fear bit by bit and learn to become comfortable with it.

This can be helpful if you suffer from anxiety and panic attacks. The main challenge here is to know whether you have general anxiety disorder or a specific phobia. In my case – general anxiety disorder – during an intake a psychologist recommended doing mindfulness instead of cognitive behavioural therapy with him.

This however is something that might be different for you, based on what you feel.

Cognitive Behavioural Therapy is a very specific form of therapy that will not be needed for all readers. I mention it because if a very specific type of fear has caused your burnout, this might be the ideal therapy for you. Plus in general, it's a therapy that helps you face your fears in a more controlled manner instead of just plunging in headfirst.

Solution: Psychotherapy (Psychiatry)

Psychotherapy or Psychiatry is the big brother of psychology that involves using medication. When your burnout is severe, medication can help greatly in countering the heavier symptoms. Being prescribed anti-depressants in combination with psychotherapy from a licensed psychiatrist will help you provide a baseline for those feelings and reverse the negative spiral.

See medication as the cushion you've landed upon to break your fall before getting up again.

Going to a psychiatrist doesn't mean you're crazy. And taking medication is not a bad thing. An acquaintance of mine followed this course for a long time after a severe depression, recovered and is now so happy it's actually kind of annoying.

However for another friend of mine, the anti-depressants didn't work at all. He turned to yoga and recovered. I guess what I'm saying is: be sure to communicate what the pills do to you with your psychiatrist, and be aware in choosing what is right for you!

If you're wondering, yes I also medicated. They were anti-anxiety drugs though and not anti-depressants. So I can't really tell you what these do to you. I just wanted to point out I feel no shame about taking medication in general.

One last tip on this subject: even if you don't need medication, but you happen to have a psychiatrist friend, contact them anyway. Having a shrink in your Help Team can be ideal! (Thank you to my dear friend Dr. Metten Somers!).

Solution: Physiotherapy and Chiropractics

Of course your mental state is also reflected in your body. As noted earlier, if you feel stressed your shoulders go up and you tense the muscles around neck, jaw and face.

Do this for a long time and you tend to get stuck. You might experience back pains or have other physical manifestations that are related to your emotional lack of wellbeing.

During my burnout I paid attention to this as well. I feel lucky I did. My lifelong friend, occasional drummer and chiropractor Martijn teamed up with physiotherapist Erik to start treating my physical symptoms in my back, neck, face and chest.

This was really, really beneficial to my recovery! So I definitely recommend looking at this as well if you experience similar manifestations.

Solution: Walking

Moving away from professional help, an amazingly simple method of recovery I'd like to discuss is simply taking a walk. Walking is one of the best solutions offered in this book, and should be added to your burnout recovery diet immediately and permanently. If you start to see walking as your baseline exercise, you will recover more quickly.

The reasons for this are numerous. Walking is a form of exercise that doesn't strain your body and is beneficial for blood flow. The forward movement also eases your mind and triggers you to think of forward moving, solution-oriented ways of improving your life. Walking also reduces cortisol levels almost instantly, and is a great in-the-moment solution to panic attacks.

Plus, walking is generally pleasant to do. It's a great way to catch up with friends, or go solo and let the surroundings sink in. It is a welcome break to your day that also burns calories and relieves aches and pains… just do it!

Solution: Music

I know what you're thinking. Walking? And now music? Really? Well, brace yourself. I'm going to give you many more unconventional solutions. They are the ones that change your mindset. Most of them, your counsellor would not even dream of giving you! But if they work, they work.

So why does music work? With music you connect all the parts of the mind that have to do with both thinking and feeling - at the same time. Your rational thoughts and your emotions merge, meaning you get rid of the discrepancies between them. Your mind literally fires up all its synapses. Your thoughts and emotions become one.

It's perfect for waking the animal.

Plus, you can choose what music to listen to. Of course, you can choose sad music, triggering you to give room to your sad emotions, or go for more aggressive music, triggering you to give room to your inner anger. You can apply this to any emotion you want to feel.

You choose the music, you choose the emotion.

On a personal note, I do recommend starting with something like reggae, slow soul music or uplifting classical music. Music that relaxes you.

(Maybe you can even look us up. Some shameless self-promotion here... check out www.earopener.com.)

And if you feel bold, try putting on James Brown's *I feel good*. You might break down and cry. But you know, try it anyway... just to see what happens ;)

Solution: Love

While we are on the subject of brain activity, let's look at love. When people are in love, brain scans show that all activity in your rational brain stops (and I mean *all*) and all the activity in the rest of the brain sparks, except for the one part responsible for our sense of fear, the amygdala.

In time, love can even make this part of the brain literally shrink.

So clinically, falling in love or loving someone reduces fear. Need I say more? Well... maybe one thing. You'll have to work out the details of this solution for yourself.

You're on your own here. Good luck.

Solution: Meditation

Meditation is another method that actually changes brain activity. It is one of the best ways to reduce your feelings of anxiety, stress, anger and depression... all negative emotions really.

So I highly recommend it, almost insisting that you pick it up. It will give immediate results too, calming your mind down and letting you get closer to what is really important from within. Classes are everywhere these days and good meditation videos are widely available online for free.

While meditation can provide instant relief, it takes longer to yield long-term results. Try to ease into it, preferably guided by a professional.

Another good reason to take it slow is that if you are not used to meditation, it can be quite confrontational. It is an inner journey. So if there is a lot of inner turmoil, you may be in for a rough ride.

In fact, meditation can make you feel worse before you feel better. It is similar to cognitive behavioural therapy because it *first* confronts you with what is wrong and makes it much more tangible. That can be a very scary process. As with CBG, it is wise to 'travel' your emotions with a guide at hand.

It took me weeks of meditation before I felt that I had made a turn for the better: on the inside that is. But on the outside, this can be different. It is likely people around you will almost immediately see a change in you when you've taken up meditation.

Your whole body and face will likely appear more relaxed to others. Even before you feel it. I've literally seen this happen to people in my meditation class. So keep meditating: what others see now is what you'll soon become.

Having said that, again, address your feelings layer by layer. See it as peeling an onion; you don't have to peel all the layers off at once. You also won't solve all your emotional challenges with meditation, despite its popularity!

Taking on challenges still requires talking and connecting with the people in your Help Team. So yes, meditate. It's great. But please don't see it as the ultimate solution. See it as another baseline.

Solution: Yoga

This is a tricky one. Yoga is regarded as one of the most beneficial practices to ease you out of a burnout. And I fully agree, it is. Plus, it will make you leaner and stronger. It's a great way to exercise. And it also forces you to let feelings flow through you without trying to change them. When you're transfixed in a pose, yoga lets you experience your feelings as they are, exactly as we discussed earlier.

But there is a catch.

Most forms of yoga involve rhythmic, controlled breathing. As a rule, it is good to mind your breathing when doing any kind of sports. And mild forms of breathing exercises can snap you out of an anxiety response.

But many of the more fanatical yoga teachers insist that yoga *is* breathing, up to the point that it becomes controlled hyperventilation.

My advice is: don't listen to them. I've been practicing yoga for a good few years now and I love it. It has also helped me with my burnout, besides making me breathe better and more consciously.

But too much of a good thing... such as *constantly* controlling your breathing, can be a double edged sword. Controlled breathing can reduce stress quickly. But if you are in a burnout, it can also trigger an anxiety response. Here too, things tend to get worse before they get better.

I've had that happen to me in class, with the constant drum of a yoga instructor saying when to breathe. It just didn't feel natural. Being conscious of how we breathe is essential. But if you're in a burnout, you should really take it easy, enjoy the benefits of controlled breathing without becoming obsessed with it.

I cannot stress this enough. You should know that I actually stopped doing yoga for a while because of this. I switched back to more aggressive sports because yoga was actually freaking me out.

This is the best example of why I'm writing this book: where most people would immediately tell you yoga is the 'greatest solution ever', I'm here to encourage you to first make up your own mind. It needs to work for you and you alone.

Basta.

So by all means, do yoga. It really, really helps to calm you down. You'll love it. But watch your step. Don't let the teachers push you too hard. Tell them you are in a burnout and they will ease you into it. Take your time and it will help you greatly. And eh… please don't turn into one of those annoying yogi types!

Solution: Breathing Exercise

Since we are talking about breathing exercises, let's focus on them specifically. Being conscious – or as they say 'mindful' – of your breathing can be very beneficial. Not just with burnout symptoms but also with recovery from all kinds of pain.

Many people breathe to the top of their lungs and don't use the full extent of their lungs by breathing into their belly. If you learn belly breathing you get more oxygen into your blood. This helps the many restorative processes in your body, including those that control your cortisol and anxiety levels.

However, here I also recommend not overdoing it. In alternative health-freak circles deep breathing is sometimes hailed as some sort of super solution to everything. And that, it definitely is not.

Furthermore, relying on breathing to snap you out of a panic attack for instance can actually make it worse if you do it the wrong way!

In the medical profession it is well known that breathing too deeply for too long actually triggers anxiety. The clinical name for it is hyperventilation.

So again, take a measured approach. A good routine could be taking a few good belly breaths, four to five times a day. There are even apps such as *Chime* that will help you remember.

You can take it further if you want. It can make a big difference for you as it did to me. But there is a right and a wrong way to do it, so consult the pros on this one - including medical professionals - and make sure you've got it right.

Solution: No More Perfectionism

It's Jedi mind trick time. In this section of our solutions, we start to look at mental practices and exercises to help you rewire your mind more quickly.

The first that I'd like to discuss is that common trigger of burnout called perfectionism, as discussed earlier.

Many of us are perfectionists. In normal situations that is fine, of course. It adds some extra 'good' pressure that can spur us into doing great things. But, always striving for perfection will always lead to things not being perfect. Even if things are going great, perfectionists tend to raise the bar even higher.

Essentially, the perfectionist keeps their personal achievement bar just out of reach. It will be forever unattainable, meaning the stress never stops. Changing your approach by scaling down the perfectionist index will prove much more useful. Not everything needs to be done at 100% capacity. You don't have to dive into everything with all you've got. In fact, a common recommendation from professionals is to switch to a 70% mode. You will find your tasks become easier to carry out and your work output improves too.

Yet saying this is easier than actually doing it. As we've shown, modern Western society can be an important factor in maintaining high stress levels by constantly bombarding us with the possibility of perfection... just before us on the horizon.

This striving for perfection is deeply ingrained in modern life. Many companies, celebrities, books and TV shows sell us on the ideal of striving for the impossible. Often they use that very word, saying things like, "*They said it was impossible, so I did it anyway.*" ... as violins start playing in the background.

We view this as inspirational and are in awe of the entrepreneurial and striving spirit behind it. Simply put, we like that kind of thinking in the Western hemisphere. But I must remind you that you are still in a burnout! Therefore you need to know that it's not the *only* way of thinking.

All cultures try to better themselves. But striving for the 'impossible' is unique to Western civilisation alone. It is always the same message: you can become better than you are right now. In essence it's an attitude problem: the bar is always put out of reach, or somewhere in the future.

The West says: "*You need to better yourself*". But the East has another message. It says: "*You are enough!*"

Solution: You are Enough

In many of the solutions we are discussing, you will be able to recognize a common theme: accepting yourself for what you are. Eastern philosophy tells us happiness comes from within and has nothing to do with achievements, let alone perfection. It's actually about the opposite: embracing your imperfections.

Countless studies show us that striving for perfection means happiness is always out of reach. This means that your cortisol levels will keep rising, which in turn negatively affects the outcome of that you are striving for. This translates into a perpetual state of unhappiness or dissatisfaction that eventually undermines your progress towards your goal.

As you'll notice from the tone of my writing, I'm particularly focused on debunking the Western myths surrounding achievement and perfectionism. While sometimes very inspirational, they are also very unattainable, and will – despite popular belief - actually have a negative impact on achieving your goals.

I am so bitter about it because it was this Western myth of achievement, innovation and perfectionism that kept me from truly reaching my goals.

It's a paradox. When I decided to let go of this perfectionist attitude and told myself I was already fine the way I was, shortly afterwards I finished an EP, an album, two books, started a new company and found love.

No joke.

Perfectionism keeps the impossible intact in your mind, thus creating stress, which in turn affects your ability to perform at an optimal level... and the cycle repeats itself. In other words, it's a myth that you can choose to believe in. I recommend you don't.

For as long as I could remember, I was a perfectionist too. But when I was finally able to break away from it, I found my stress levels went down almost overnight. I realized that striving for the perfect is a useless distraction that actually prevents you from ever coming close to it.

Instead of automatically reaching for a goal on the distant horizon, first go within yourself and embrace what you already have to work with. And then find out later, if your output was perfect or not.

This does not mean you can't dream of things being better or strive for things that can enhance your life and your happiness. Of course you can! Those desires are part of what is within you.

Just remember to keep them separate in your mind. Let yourself move towards goals without striving for perfection. Accepting who you are is the key.

It's a paradox that many of us in the West still find hard to accept. But you are in a burnout, and so you must. Being at peace with all your imperfections will give you clarity on how to achieve the goals you set for yourself.

That is why Eastern philosophies always start with repeating something: you already have everything you need to achieve greatness. It's not somewhere on the horizon, it's all within you.

You are enough.

Solution: Thankfulness and Forgiveness

Staying on this theme, you can also train your mind to be more grateful and forgiving about your life in general. It's a radical change of mindset, and heart. You start by telling yourself you are enough. And that you are thankful for the things that are good in your life, and you forgive yourself and others for their mistakes and their imperfections.

I realize this sounds like higher Buddha doctrine. And some of you reading this will probably feel uncomfortable with this solution. So did I. I thought doing this would turn me into a squishy little yogi with his head permanently in the clouds. So I hate to tell you this...

...it works (sorry)! And for your information, I have not turned into a wimp! But still, I'm happy to make it a little less 'yogi' and a lot more practical as a solution for you to incorporate in your recovery routine:

Try to write down one thing every day that you feel good about. Doesn't matter what - big or small. This will help get your feet back on the ground by reminding you of the good things already in your life.

Granted, it's a bite size solution (a thousand tiny steps)... but there are some heftier solutions just around the corner in the same vein as Thankfulness.

Solution: Visualization & Neuro Linguistics

This Thankfulness approach lays the groundwork for a Jedi mind trick that can be even more effective. We can discuss two methods at the same time here: Visualization and Neuro Linguistic Programming.

The technique of Visualization teaches us to visualize where we want to be and how we want to feel. It makes our dreams more tangible to us.

The theory goes that the more you visualize a desired outcome, the closer you get to your goal because you will automatically and subconsciously do the things that get you there. This concept has helped many people achieve their dreams.

The catch is of course to not visualize things being too perfect! Again my advice here is that when you want to use this technique, take a measured approach.

The same can be said about the technique of Neuro Linguistic Programming. This method involves you telling yourself – through language – the things you want to be and repeating them as often as needed for it to become true. It is quite a useful technique in burnout circumstances because subtle changes in language can have big effects.

Let me give you an example. Instead of telling yourself you *are* stressed, you can tell yourself you are *acting* stressed. This makes all the difference in the world. If you 'are' stressed, it is something that is 'in a state of being' and you can't change it. But if you 'act' stressed, it is not something that 'is' and you can change it this very instant.

Just stop acting stressed.

The benefits of both Visualization and Neuro Linguistic Programming go beyond burnout recovery and bring you into the realm of reaching your full potential. Just try to separate the Western and Eastern approach.

The Western approach tells us we can become more than we actually are. If you visualize or linguistically program yourself to this idea of success, you will increase stress because achieving it remains out of reach. The Eastern approach tells us we are already enough. If you visualize or linguistically program yourself to this perspective, you will be more open to creating your own success.

One tactic says you have to change something or add something in order to be complete. The other tells you that you are already complete, and in the process of becoming more yourself - the person you already are.

Which one do you think is better for your self-esteem and overall stress levels?

Solution: Mindfulness

Acceptance of ourselves and an increased awareness of our inner psyche are also the basis for a relatively new and increasingly popular meditation practice called Mindfulness.

What this practice teaches us is to be aware of what we are feeling *in the moment*. It doesn't provide solutions or prescribe answers per se (so it's not the same as going to a psychologist!). But it does provide the clarity we need to get to a solution.

Basically, you become aware of an emotion and label it as just that - an emotion. When you do this, you can examine what this emotion does to you physically and mentally. With this knowledge, you'll become better at choosing how to respond to this emotion.

Let's take the emotion of fear again, to provide us with an example. With mindfulness training, you become aware or mindful that you are experiencing the emotion fear. All of a sudden, you can be more analytical about that emotion. You can 'assess' what it does to you. You can ask yourself the question: why am I fearful when I'm standing in line at the grocery store?

If this all sounds like more higher Buddha science, don't fret. It's fundamentally the same idea as counting to ten when you feel something. Instead of immediately starting to cry or behaving in a very angry way, you take a step back. You learn to let the emotions flow through you, to recognize what's going on, and become more mindful of when and how to respond or perhaps not respond.

The primary meditation that is used is called the 'body-scan'. In this meditation, you mentally go from toe to pinkie finger and through all your other body parts to see *how they feel*. In the meantime, your mind starts to drift.

What Mindfulness gives you is the experience of mental drifting and then returning your focus on your body.

The effect is that you become more aware of the moment – the now - instead of always drifting away to your burnout related thoughts about the future or the past. The ultimate trick for reversing burnout is that you start to recognize when your mind is building up doomsday scenarios that aren't actually there - and recognize when thoughts are not facts.

For instance, you learn to see that a lot of your anxiety is just a scary movie playing itself out in your mind. And like a scary movie, it isn't real. Mindfulness can help you to distinguish simulation from reality. You learn when the emotions you feel are useful, and when not.

I found this practice very helpful, even enjoyable. But I also found you should limit yourself and install a cap on just how far you want to go in this. If you dive too deeply, you'll start to overanalyze all your emotions, which is the opposite of what you should be doing!

For those of you suffering from panic attacks, it is very, very helpful, but also recommended to take it slow. Remember, putting focus on the panic is what causes the panic in the first place. Be 'mindful' of that!

To those of you who suffer from trauma and/or PTSD I also highly recommend it. Mindfulness stops the process of re-experiencing the trauma in your mind. It brings you in connection with your surroundings in the now, thus stopping the memory from manifesting itself.

So try out mindfulness. It worked for me. But do so with the cause of your burnout firmly in mind. You can later decide if it should be part of your baseline. And make sure you stay deeply connected to your inner animal as well.

Solution: Tai Chi (Chuan)

While Mindfulness is one of the youngest of the Eastern philosophy based techniques, Tai Chi is one of the oldest. However, they have the same effect - they both put you in the moment, calm your mind and refocus your energy. Tai Chi is also the best bridge from mental practices to physical exercises in this solution-focused chapter.

I love Tai Chi. Not only is it the first step towards Kung Fu, it is also simply beautiful to witness. For those of you who have problems getting your energy levels up, Tai Chi is your go-to practice. Plenty of free instruction videos are also available online, so there is nothing stopping you.

The beauty of Tai Chi is that it doesn't take any energy to begin with. It is based on super-slow movements that are effortless. But when you're done, your energy will be renewed. It's a paradox: the slow movements build up energy.

There is a second benefit as well. Tai Chi is very good for muscle development. Working your muscles is a sure method to reduce burnout symptoms. But while some of you probably have no interest in hitting the gym right now, Tai Chi is an ideal option that eases you into muscle development. It builds them back up from the core.

Another benefit to Tai Chi is its silence. Unlike many meditations, yoga practices or mindfulness teachings, it doesn't rely on talking you through it. You just watch and follow the movement. It is meditative in itself without all the fluff that tends to come with its new age cousins. And that's refreshing by definition.

Plus... Tai Chi is 1500 years old, and translates to *Supreme Ultimate Boxing.*

So badass. Do it.

Solution: Cardio & Weight Training

While we are on the subject of muscle development, let's move away from developing mindsets and into the subject of exercise.

Physical exercise is always recommended, even when you're not in a burnout situation. It's beneficial for just about everything: preventing diseases, your overall mood, your work ethic... you name it. So play some tennis or soccer or whatever your game is. If anything, it will set your mind on something other than your burnout! Take it easy of course... but have fun.

You should know that for your recovery, there are some differences between cardio and weight training. Cardio is good exercise and will make you feel better. But weight training will help you recover more quickly because it specifically increases testosterone that reduces cortisol levels in the muscle recovery phase.

So, although both cardio and weight training are useful, you may benefit more from weight training.

As with perfection, I recommend going only 70% on exercise. Don't wear yourself out completely because you'll need your energy for other things. Make it a regular part of your regime, instead of going all-out and having to take time to recover afterwards. Be energy mindful!

It is worth noting that people can become even more stressed out by overtraining. It is fine to push yourself to better your overall physical condition. But if exercising or working out becomes obsessive, it can be one of the more pronounced burnout triggers.

So easy does it.

Solution: Stop Running

There is one type of training that deserves special mention: running. You can go out running or jogging if you really think it is best – it's your personal recovery and one hundred percent your choice – but for the record: I don't recommend it.

In fact almost everyone, from my general practitioner to my trainer to the psychiatrist who helped me write this book, told me: *"... just as long as you don't go out running"*.

And they might be right. Running not only puts enormous stress on our leg muscles and joints taking impact after impact on hard surfaces, it also raises our cortisol levels more quickly than other forms of exercise, especially for those of us past forty years old.

Minutes into the run our body starts to produce large amounts of cortisol... and we know what that means.

Let me give you a case where running was actually the cause of stress. A girl I know had become so obsessed with marathon running that in the end, her boyfriend told her that he would pay for her Mindfulness training if she just... stopped... running.

Also, I suffered my second major anxiety attack during a run, just after I reached that coveted 'runner's high'. I just thought you should know that.

Solution: Boxing, Martial Arts and Game-Sports

A special shout out in the exercise department goes to boxing and other forms of contact sports or martial arts. I'm a lifelong boxer myself and can tell you these types of sports demand a higher amount of physical control than other sports. Because if you don't use control, someone could get hurt!

Aside from the fact that for professional martial artists punching someone is kind of the point, the emphasis on controlling your body and your aggression wakes up the inner animal. It gets you out of the burnout mindset.

Plus practicing martial arts relieves you of your feelings of anger that, despite what many may think, are just as much a part of burnout as the other emotions we have discussed.

The same can be said about sports involving strategy and/or hand-eye coordination. Sports like tennis, soccer, and squash take your mind away from your burnout because of the focused concentration involved. This relieves symptoms – and as we discussed – might even be enough for some of you to fast forward your recovery.

Solution: Dancing, Singing, Massages, Sex...

Of course the ultimate physical contact is the loving and caring contact we have with others. It should come as no surprise that kissing and sex are probably the best cortisol reducers and 'good' hormone enhancers there are.

But if you have no sexual partner at this time, or sex is not really on your mind, a simple hug can already do wonders. Booking a massage or a physiotherapy session is another good way to relieve stress.

Or, just go dancing. Or take singing lessons.

Exercise, martial arts, sex, dancing, singing... and in the same vein, saunas, stretching, and massages get you 'out of your mind and into your body'. Your burnout is mental *and* emotional. It forms in your mind and has an effect on your body. When you concentrate on just the body, the mind immediately starts to ease up.

Solution: Acupuncture

Deliberately focussing on your body is one method. There are also ways to spark your body into healing itself without you deliberately focussing on it. One of those methods is acupuncture.

This Chinese-based alternative medical practice identifies pressure points around the body that have an effect on other parts of your body and even your mind. In acupuncture sticking tiny needles into them activates these points!

I wish I could tell you that this solution really is too far out (think of it - needles!), but I can't. It really works. Don't ask me how. All I know is there are pressure points that can increase your intake of oxygen, relieve pain, and really calm you down.

This is an ancient method that millions upon millions of practitioners have perfected over the millennia. Keep an open mind, and it can work for you too.

What it does is wondrous. It activates areas of your body to heal themselves within days. And the funny thing is, you won't notice it...until you do.

All of a sudden, you don't feel that ache anymore. All of a sudden, you are more relaxed than you thought you would be. It even helps the body deal with addictions. All of a sudden, days after the treatment, you don't want to smoke anymore. Or, you don't feel like drinking. It's nothing less than magic!

Solution: Binaural Beats

Acupuncture is as old as binaural beats are new. These are wavelengths of sound, often merged with relaxing music, that have a subconscious effect similar to acupuncture.

When you listen to binaural beats (you can easily find them online), your body goes into a state of healing that at first you will not notice, but will later have a positive effect on your state of mind, and can relieve headaches and similar stress related pains.

I do recommend taking it slow though. It's one gigantic mystery really that involves brain waves and can be a little uncomfortable. Yet binaural beats have been proven to alleviate feelings of tension in the mind and the body.

Solution: Change Your Diet (Part I)

Talking about the body - and getting down to basics - this next solution may also surprise some of you: change your diet! Sugars, meat, too many carbohydrates and the wrong kind of fats found in processed food all heighten your stress levels.

Starting with sugars, these are almost instantly taken up in your blood. Your body is designed to burn your food and transform it into natural sugars to give you energy. But when you ingest sugars directly, your body goes into a particular kind of survival mode, tricking it into thinking it can get the energy right now and making it crave even more. Hence, that whole package of cookies you somehow *need* to finish.

Because of this instant effect, you become hungry again quickly after eating sugars. The cycle then repeats itself so that you run the risk of your body only wanting more sugar. Constant feelings of hunger linger, bringing you more stress while your body grows bigger, and your energy is depleted. In essence, this is stress induced by sugar imbalances.

Carbohydrates found in rice, potatoes and wheat-based products are better energy 'bringers' than sugars because they deliver the sugars found in them in a more gradual manner. Too much of these however, means your stomach needs to do a lot of work. This means your energy levels will be further depleted. For many of us, this loss of energy can be enough to trigger sombreness and a feeling of constant fatigue.

The same process can be experienced when digesting processed food, especially salty snacks. Not only will these deplete your energy levels, but also they are likely to trigger blood and heart related conditions that in turn, increase anxiety.

Last, but not least, is meat. Many of the so called 'healthy' diets these days focus on eating lots of proteins that are naturally found in meats. Animal based proteins however are notoriously hard to digest, much harder than foods such as fruits, vegetables and nuts, and can take hours longer to process.

But that is not the only thing to consider when eating meat. Animals are slaughtered, leaving stress hormones in the meat that you eat. In a way, you are taking in small portions of their stress, just before they were put down. These hormones enter your blood flow, quite literally increasing your cortisol levels.

There are millions of people who have at least temporarily changed their diet when they suffered from burnout. For some of you, the diet will not be the problem if you already have a healthy and balanced diet. And, there is also the consideration that changing your diet is challenging, and you may not want to add another stress factor to your regime right now.

So, forgive yourself for those cookies, and then consider what changing your diet could do for you. You'd be amazed what a vegetarian diet can do to reduce stress levels. It is worth pursuing, even if only for a limited period of time. Plus, it will make you feel better and more in touch with your body, which can be a huge boost to self-esteem.

Solution: Change Your Diet (Part II)

While a change of diet benefits the great majority of people, it is worth noting that it can also work the other way around. For those of you who are on a strict vegan diet and still suffer burnout symptoms: go grab a big steak, some ice cream or a bag of chips right now!

Healthy eating is a huge trend in modern societies. However for some, it has become a craze with potentially dire consequences.

In my own circle, I've seen three cases of women who became so strict in their vegan diets that they lost way too much weight. You can see this one coming a mile away... eating too little or too strictly *greatly* increases stress levels. It sends the cortisol through the roof because your entire being is craving the energy it's not getting!

In one case, a lady friend of mine had to be hospitalized. The doctors told her she was on the brink of collapse or worse because she had been a strict vegan for years. The advice they gave her? Quit being vegan and stop stressing about food.

In short, you are what you eat. Be mindful, it helps. But please don't overdo it! You can change your diet for the better, but don't go *on* a diet. Don't stress over food. That will only make things worse.

Solution: Magnesium and Other Supplements

Even when you change your diet, sometimes your body still needs a little help. Vitamin supplements, such as magnesium and turmeric (curcuma longa), irons, vitamin C or B, are often recommended in cases of burnout because they are natural stress reducers and inhibitors. Specialised supplements containing valerian do the same, and have an added benefit: you sleep better.

Supplements can drive away symptoms, not causes. But when your symptoms subside, you will feel better equipped to deal with the causes of your burnout. Again, I recommend not leaning too heavily on this as a single solution. A healthy diet can be supplemented, but supplements are not enough to make up for an unhealthy diet.

Still, I have found supplements worth experimenting with. Magnesium can be very beneficial, and even serve as a muscle relaxant. So beneficial in fact that, because I hadn't been able to relax for such a long time during my burnout, when I experienced the calming effects of magnesium, I almost freaked out!

Solution: Kicking the Habit

On the subject of freaking out, be aware that alcohol, drugs, nicotine and the like all instantly heighten your stress levels. Kicking these habits can greatly reduce your burnout symptoms. We tend to think it is the other way around, that this glass of wine or that cigarette is what gives us comfort. But in fact, the comfort is only short-lived and they soon become triggers.

I'll make this short and sweet. Get professional help if you can't kick these habits alone. And of course, don't beat yourself up if you can't beat them instantly. Don't be too harsh on yourself. Almost everyone around you has something they need to quit or mitigate somehow. And remember, people recover by changing habits that hold them back - from themselves.

Solution: Keeping a Diary

Moving away from the body, let's look at some other practical behavioural changes that work for the better. An excellent tip is to write both your positive and negative emotions down *at* the time you experience them.

Keeping a diary is a proven method in helping you understand what you are going through. Log the times, how you feel, on what scale your emotions were felt, why you think you felt them, where you were and exactly what you were feeling. Then reread your notes the next day.

This helps to keep burnout in perspective. It shows you that you've gone through bad times and come out on the other side.

And there is another good reason to do this. You can reread it when you've recovered, reminding yourself to keep taking things easy even when you are not suffering from burnout, and to again feel proud that you have recovered.

Solution: Stop Multitasking and Disconnect

This solution will not come as a surprise to you, I hope. Constant multitasking or being online all the time increases stress levels. Both serve as distractions from your work-life balance that in time can get the better of you.

Multitasking has been proven to be a complete and utter myth. Having technology around us hasn't magically changed our physiology. Countless research studies have debunked this myth. When we divide our attention over multiple sources, we drift off and forget to be mindful of the moment. It's a sure trigger to generalized anxiety.

Of course, this suggestion is only meant to reduce symptoms. But as we've shown, drowning out the noise that is constantly available is a pivotal part of your recovery. Take breaks, a walk, get some fresh air, or disconnect, and don't put all those screens on at the same time!

Solution: Stop Procrastinating

Ok, I know you are raising an eyebrow right now, but I'm really serious. Procrastination is actually a very common cause of burnout. It's one of those things we do that makes us wallow in our minds - frozen in our burnout. In the book, *The War of Art* by Steven Pressfield, it's called 'creative resistance', and it goes like this:

Most of us have creative dreams. In fact, most readers of this book have some sort of creative challenge that calls to them. But when in burn out, we all face resistance in picking up on the goals we have set out for ourselves.

Most creative people know that *doing* the task at hand is not the hard part, whereas *starting* it is. We all have excuses that stop us from achieving our goals. Take your pick - first doing the laundry, watching some TV, taking some time off to think, going out with friends, waiting for 'inspiration', or jumping into the shower.

Another option is feeling sorry for ourselves for whatever reason... or my personal favourite go-to procrastination scenario: making very long 'to do' lists (which by the way, I recommend you stop doing immediately).

In and of itself, procrastinating is not a bad thing. Setting distractions for ourselves can give us new ideas. It's a funny trick of the mind: we get the best ideas while doing something completely unrelated. In fact, we need to procrastinate from time to time to let our mind release more of our creativity.

However, if you are pushing the task away for days, weeks, months or even years, it means you will start to feel a very particular kind of stress: the stress that you have failed in achieving or pursuing your dreams. It makes you feel you're wasting your life. Can you see the burnout on the horizon before you?

This sense of 'I've failed in my life' is one of the worst types of anxiety there is. Eventually, this stress will break you down. Believe me, I've been there!

The burnout symptom that is most closely linked to this is sleep anxiety: afraid you will fall asleep and not wake up. Once you have experienced this symptom, it becomes hard to break away from it. And simply because of a lack of sleep, you experience even more tension and anxiety during the night.

There is a cure. One that I advise adopting this very moment: Start. Your. Project... even if it means putting down this book! This type of anxiety will not go away unless you take action. It's a cliché that's very true. You can change your life for the better in literally one second by just getting started with the task or dream you have set for yourself!

This will put you on the path of your dreams, and relieve your generalized anxiety. It's the type of work that creates calm within instead of increasing stress. If you recognize this as a possible cause to your burnout, I recommend starting, continuing or – always the hardest part - finishing your life project now.

You may also want to do some research into procrastination by reading The War of Art, or talking about your journey with fellow creators. Most likely you will feel the most stress building up when you're doing your project, but it's *good* stress - the type that makes you excited and energetic!

In short, if procrastination is your burnout cause, I'm telling you to buck up, put your best foot forward, and simply get started.

Solution: Work on love

And this procrastination thing goes beyond creative projects. If you procrastinate about your love life and constantly dwell on a muddy past or impossible expectations, you will not find love. While love is a fantastic anxiety reducer!

There is a simple solution that you can put in motion right now: take action. Move on. Find a date, or talk to the loved one you have trouble connecting with.

It doesn't matter how, just as long as you stop procrastinating and start doing *something*.

Procrastinating in love is something we all do. We're conditioned to think of love as something that will magically come to us in a perfect form, and then - dreaming away - we marry and live happily ever after.

Yet feeling happy is something that is already happening inside of you, and not only experienced on a date or with your partner. All of us who have had love in our lives know that with experience, we become better at it.

Whether it's love, sports, creative projects, careers... or whatever we dream of, the trick is to just start believing, doing something about it and building up experience that we learn from.

In certain cases, it can also be about letting go of certain dreams. Procrastinating about things that will never become a reality is just as bad as postponing tangible dreams that are clearly possible. It's about acceptance, letting go and then picking up the things you *can* do.

Now. This *second*.

Solution: Don't Believe in The Law of Attraction

Before we wind up our solution chapter, there is something I'd like to address in this final part: a solution that doesn't work. It is a mindset solution that falls firmly in the category of Jedi mind tricks. It is called the Law of Attraction and is very similar to Visualisation and Neuro Linguistic Programming: you attract that which you think about.

We have already covered such mindset methods and know they can work to improve your frame of mind, and reduce negative thoughts that translate into stressed out bodies. So there is nothing wrong with the Law of Attraction perspective at face value! However, I must issue a warning when you combine this idea with your burnout symptoms.

This is a very particular and quite popular 'cure' making the rounds on the Internet - the very enthusiastic 'guru' types who tell you that the solution to your burnout is to keep saying to yourself that you don't have a burnout.

This is of course very dangerous.

While the Law of Attraction can be powerful under non-burnout circumstances, I do not recommend making it specifically about your burnout. Believing in this solution has a very cruel catch. If you keep repeating to yourself that you are fine while clearly you are not, it will backfire.

You must accept you are not fine and give yourself time to recover.

I'm sorry that this solution doesn't work. But unfortunately, you can't mind control yourself out of everything...

Solution: A Holiday

All right, we've reached the last solution I have to offer: taking a holiday.

It can help.

Just don't think a holiday will solve burnout.

You can run, but you can't hide from your inner feelings. They are always with you, no matter where you are. So don't take a holiday if it is only about running away. Take it if you think it will help give some more clarity.

Also, don't expect too much from a vacation for the same reasons. You're still on an inner journey. Go, enjoy and keep your recovery expectations in check and you'll be one step closer to recovery.

So yes. Take one. Rest and then recover.

Part V: Rising up Again

How Your Recovery Will Feel

Hopefully one of the solutions I've presented, or a combination or variation thereof, is helping you get back on your feet. You are recovering of course, but chances are that while you're reading this, you haven't fully recovered yet. So I'd like to use this last part of the book to manage some of your expectations and prepare you for the journey still ahead.

Here I can only speak from personal experience. I've had a lot of fallbacks, and I mean a *lot*. There were countless times I felt I wasn't improving, or even that my condition was getting worse. At the time, I hadn't realized that feeling worse was the result of letting go of my emotions. In this way, feeling bad was actually a good thing.

What basically happens is... your emotions are coming back to life. That's good but there is a catch. Although finally really *feeling* again is fantastic, those emotions do tend to be a little out of control in this period of the recovery. And by little I mean a lot.

I had intense, uncontrollable anger outburst. My punching bag still hates me deeply. Fear felt different too. Instead of dreading it, I started to... how do I put this... *enjoy* fear. I could finally recognize the use of fear: it was telling me where the edge was. And showing me whether or not I could cross those boundaries.

And sometimes the experience of feeling joy was so fresh to me – I hadn't felt that for so long – I broke down and cried. It must have been one hell of a peculiar sight to behold: during these intense waterfalls that were just crushing down from my eyes, I would yell to my loved ones how great I felt.

Weird as hell man.

It was just so strange to feel happiness again. You are essentially faking it until you make it. You just keep pushing those emotions out and somewhere along the line they will balance out again.

You will also start to look much better before you feel better. This is weird too. I had moments I still felt like utter crap while somebody was paying me a compliment on just how healthy I looked.

And things tend to get worse before they get better. It came as a shock to me just how much emotional upkeep I had neglected. It is likely you will experience similar feelings and situations. In those moments it is important to remember that it's all for a good cause. Plus, remember to contact your Help Team if and when you feel this way.

That emotional fog *will* lift. You will walk around feeling numb yet knowing that you will start to feel great again at some point. And you will. For sure.

But even after reading all of the above, if you are really still feeling down, don't worry. I've held back on one important insight - just for this moment - that could help you immensely. The last piece of advice I can give you that could tip the burnout recovery balance in your favour: *Care less.* Yes, you're reading this right.

Care. Less.

How to Care a Little Less

During a burnout so many of us get preoccupied with thoughts and emotions about three things: what happened in the past, what's happening now and what could happen in the future. It can be really hard to let go of those thoughts, even when we have no control over what happened, is happening or could still happen.

Learning to take distance and consider these thoughts and the emotions that come with them will most certainly help you recover. It will make you aware of how your thoughts can steer your emotions. So yes, you absolutely need to work on that. Everyone will tell you this: teach yourself not to emotionally dwell on the things you can't control.

Be that as it may, sometimes you'll still feel like nothing can help you out of this mess. You can't help but dwell. But thankfully there is still one card up your sleeve that could help you big time in the direst of moments: Stoicism.

When the feelings become too overwhelming the philosophy of Stoicism can steady the storm. It teaches us that nothing is good or bad and everything is just what it is. In other words: it teaches us not to judge everything - all the time.

It's an ancient Greek philosophy that has been practiced by many of the most successful people on earth. It is all about acceptance and deliberately choosing how you feel about something, or even choosing simply not to give a damn.

That's right, it tells you *feeling emotion can be a choice.*

Let's see how this works. Maybe you feel really bad about a political situation, a career that has failed or any of the other triggers and causes we have discussed on these pages. Maybe you wish you could change the past. Maybe you are anxious about what other people think about you right now. Or maybe you worry about the future a lot.

These dwellings create feelings, and the emotions that come up in that moment need to flow through you as valuable signals. But however valuable they may be, those negative emotions still bring you a lot of hurt, sadness or anxiety when you experience them. And when you're really down, really sick and tired of dealing with a burnout... well, try something else for a change:

To not give a fuck.

Emotions are a choice

Now I've told you to embrace your inner animal, which you really should. You need to get to the bottom of those emotions. But you are still capable of rational thought. So when the beast is making you too emotional and it becomes too much to bare… switch back to the rational mode.

A great way to do this is by being stoic about something. Feel hurt? So what. Everybody feels hurt sometimes. Feel anxious? Why should I? It's not bringing me anything. Feel like your country is going to hell in a hand basket under the new president? You know what, you can't change any of it. So why should you care?

Indeed. Why *should* you care? Should you care about *everything*? The answer is of course no. You don't have to carry the world on your shoulders, especially when your needs are closer to home.

Learning how your emotional signals work in your body and mind gives you the tools to change them. It creates the opportunity to change what you feel. So instead of feeling bad because you're say, grumpy… you change that feeling into being happy about being grumpy.

Just let yourself be bloody grumpy and feel bloody good about it.

Being stoic doesn't work in all cases of course. And I'd hate to think you'd become a cold indifferent person. But you'd be surprised to find out just how effective it can be.

So what if you have a burnout. It happens to the strong, not the weak. So what if that career is ending. You can build a new one, just like you did the old. So what if you're late. So what if you don't feel like going out. Who cares what people post on social media. So bloody what.

Don't become careless. But do care less.

Pick out the things you should care about, the things you can control. And become more stoic about the things you can let go of. Don't focus too much on them. Make your choice and choose your battles.

Must, Can and Wish

A good way to help you make choices about what to really care about comes from a trick Brigitte taught me. When you are faced with a choice you can slice it up in three ways. Must I do it? Can I do it? Or, do I really wish to do it?

There are a lot of things we *can* do in our lives. But this doesn't mean we *must* do them or we *want or wish* to do them. Other things are *wishes* we have. But it doesn't mean we *can* reach them. Still other things *must* be done. But that doesn't mean we'll enjoy doing them.

This distinction can be hugely important. It's linguistic programming. Many of us use the word 'must' more often than we use 'can' or 'wish'. We say: "I must do my work" instead of "I can" or "I want to", or an even a milder variation like "I should" or "I'd like to", or the stoic answer "I will".

The choice of words can make all the difference. If you constantly tell yourself you *must* do everything, you'll start to resist it and become more stressed out sooner or later. You'll start to feel everything is a 'must' and nothing is a choice ('can') or something enjoyable ('wish').

In a burnout, there is very little you should feel obliged to do. Very few true *musts*. But there are a huge amount of things you *can* do to get out of it. Probably there are even a lot of things you *want* to do because you know they will make you feel better.

So getting out of the burnout is a lot about *can/wish* and very little about *must*. It's not that you must go to the psychologist or book that massage. But you can do it or can wish to do it. It's a choice. A choice you control.

When you start using the right words, you make possibility part of your subconscious. You will develop a 'can do' attitude.

Reclaiming Lust for Life

And yes you can. You can get back into the fray of modern life. At first, it will feel very strange being happy again. You'll even feel uncomfortable because it's been such a long time since you felt that kind of happiness. You'll have changed. So it'll be a new experience picking up your life again.

Yet this time you'll be much better prepared. You have learned who you are from the inside. You know with one hundred percent certainty when to say no and when not to care because your gut will tell you. You have integrated a lot of good behaviour into your life, from better diets to more exercise, love and relaxation.

Your energy has returned and the path ahead of you will be easier and clearer. You've reclaimed your lust for life. You can now see your career in a better perspective. No more swimming up river - just you, going with the flow.

Your shoulders will hang lower and your belly will stick out just a little bit more from belly breathing. And you don't really care about that. Your inner animal has taught you that not everything the world throws at you is worth pursuing and not all relationships are created equal.

Work doesn't engulf your entire life anymore. Nor does social media or whatever crisis all those oversized egos in politics have just concocted. Plus, you've learned to put away that Smartphone when you are with people you can connect with.

You've drowned out the noise. You're back in control. You know when to listen to your thoughts or when they are just passing signals and emotions not worth going after.

You've lowered your expectations and have lost the need for perfection. In return, you've gained the insights you needed to achieve what you want.

Plus, you've learned to acknowledge the right and the wrong kind of stress. You have embraced the opportunity of your burnout, turned it into a victory, strengthening yourself and your relationships with loved ones.

And pretty soon you'll find yourself explaining to others what they can do to get out of their stressful situation.

And even though you still face many challenges in your life, you now feel much better equipped to deal with them than ever before.

Those burned out tires have been replaced. Your phoenix has risen and your butterfly has emerged from its cocoon.

You've broken down to the break through.

You are reborn. You are whole. You are enough.

Welcome to your restart.

Extra's

The Panic Trick

As promised in the beginning of the book, I've added this chapter for those suffering from panic attacks as I have. It's about learning to recognize and deal with them using the so-called *panic trick*, as David Carbonell calls it in his *Panic Attacks Workbook* (which again, I highly recommend reading!).

The good news is that panic attacks are one hundred percent curable. They can literally vanish. The bad news is that if you are reading this extra chapter you are still suffering from them. Hence, you haven't found the right way to deal with them yet. Fortunately, once you understand the trick, the panic can go away. So what is this panic trick? It goes like this:

When you think about panic, you will start to panic.

Usually, the first panic attack you get is the worst. This attack has a very clear function; it's the first time your body has signalled your need to become a couch potato for a while. My first heart palpitations, landing me in the emergency room at the hospital, came five years prior to the burnout itself. Maybe I should've listened more carefully back then…

I've had many attacks since. And panic attacks truly are horrific. From feeling like you are having a heart attack, to feeling you will faint or need to throw up or even feeling totally detached from the world… panic attacks are like tornados ripping through your chest and the very core of your being. Cortisol levels go up, reach a climax… and then it's all over. And you're fine again.

Panic attacks became so frequent for me that I developed a general anxiety disorder. The cruel irony is that the later attacks serve much less of a function than the first. They occur for one simple reason: you don't want to ever experience them again. So when you get into situations where your stress levels might go up, you start to think: I don't want to have a panic attack. Not now. I don't want it. Stop! And then it hits you bigtime.

Your focus on the attack makes the panic *rise* instead of fall. You remember how it feels. You start to obsess over it. The last time you thought you were going to throw up. So now you're thinking about throwing up. And then you think: what if this time I really do throw up? And before you know it, you really feel like throwing up. It's a vicious cycle.

Even if feeling sick to your stomach or other symptoms don't occur during all of your panic attacks, the fear that they will becomes so strong that you can't stop yourself from anticipating the worst. That thinking ultimately induces the attack.

And you run. You get out of the situation you're in. And when the panic goes down, you assure yourself: running was the right thing to do. Or you develop other countermeasures and rationalisations to counter the attack. Carbonell divides these into: *Avoidance, Protective Rituals, Superstitions, Support People or Objects*. These countermeasures could be having a certain pill handy to calm you when you go out, or having someone standing by on speed dial.

The problem is that all those countermeasures serve as a constant reminder that you are suffering from panic attacks… thus reminding you of them at any time… and in turn, inducing more panic attacks. Even worse, the more you cling to countermeasures, the worse your panic attacks will become. So you need to find a way to go on with your life without those constant reminders!

Now I'm not saying that you can't use things that can help. I've had many things that helped, including a small bag of lavender that I would sniff to help calm me down. What I am saying is that the countermeasures must not become a permanent part of your daily rituals. If they do, these countermeasures will actually *cause* more panic attacks.

To recover from the anxiety disorder, I first had to reduce the triggers and then just accept the symptoms as they came to me during panic attacks. I had to learn not to do anything when the attack came and just let it flow through me. In time, I learned the attacks always go away. This meant I stopped thinking about them.

I also had to confront myself with the situations that sparked the attacks. If you keep ignoring them, things will also get worse. Psychologists call this *to desensitize*. The more you let yourself experience that uncomfortable situation, the easier it will be to reduce panic because you have become more desensitized to the trigger.

But most of all, I had to start seeing panic attacks for the trick that they really are. That's what ultimately freed me of them.

Assembling The Help Team

Assembling The Help Team will of course be highly personal to you. I've added this extra chapter so you can read about my Help Team, just to give you some extra inspiration when you are assembling yours. Also, it is a way for me to thank them again. This chapter acknowledges all the puzzle pieces that the people on a Help Team can represent, and how they make up the entire finished puzzle.

This book came about with the help of a brilliant psychiatrist and my good friend Metten Somers, who runs the Psych Ward of a large hospital and has experience with the worst of mental problems. My problem was not severe enough for me to need a psychiatrist. However, talking to such an experienced professional gave me so much perspective. I really welcomed it and if you know someone who can do the same, I highly recommend tapping into that resource. Plus in the process, Metten and I became even closer friends.

A special shout out goes to Kerim Fathallah, my mindfulness teacher. He brought wisdom and expertise into the team on how to deal with everyday life. Plus he encouraged me to play music much more than I was before. He immediately recognised this was a great way for me to express my emotions and not overthink things.

My main helper in my recovery was a genius haptotherapist, Carolien van Dijk. She took my emotional turmoil seriously but also stayed very grounded. Her down to earth attitude made me feel very safe. I guess what I'm saying here is that having someone in the Help Team who is grounded, really helps.

Of course I was greatly helped by people who can focus on the physical side of burnout, like trainers, coaches, physiotherapists... the lot. Keep those who can help you with strengthening your body as close as possible!

I've had a lot of help from my family too. Once they had grasped the severity of the situation, they refrained from judgement. They did give me gentle nudges here and there. But the important thing for you to remember is that it can really help to have some people who don't have to necessarily have to do anything, but are simply there for you.

Two of my best female friends Lauren Verster and Anne Schipper were there for me as my speed dial helpers. Especially with anxiety attacks, they were the ones keeping me grounded. My male friends (my old homies) were there at a distance. I didn't feel like contacting them all the time, but having that beer together every once in awhile… was priceless.

Brigitte Kalkhoven… where do I begin? I found her in my worst moment, gave her a very hard time and she still stayed with me - even in the moments when she couldn't.

The last mention is to you, my readers. I don't know you but writing to you has been a big help. So thank you for playing an unwitting role as part of my Help Team.

And if you wish to connect, remember to pay a visit to www.restart-burnout-book.com. Or check out our music at www.earopener.com.

I wish you a speedy recovery!

Lessons I've learned and other useful thoughts

- You are enough
- You are not alone
- Burnout is the worlds' number one affliction
- People recover, restart and feel reborn
- You can make it highly personal
- The way into a burnout is not the same as out
- Negative emotions are ok, they're part of life
- Everyone gets depressed at least once in life
- Surrender is often a winning tactic
- Stress builds up but also goes down
- It's not a giant leap but a thousand tiny steps
- Burnout happens to the strong, not the weak
- Letting go of pride makes you feel awesome
- Sometimes it's enough to just lower expectations
- Don't *get* happy, just *be* happy
- The power of your mind is great
- It's nice to drown out the noise
- Focus on everything you *can* control
- Striving for perfection prevents achieving it
- Write down one good thing a day
- Don't say you *are* stressed, say you *act* stressed
- Stay in the now
- Walk. Train. Stretch. Move. Repeat.
- Dance. Sing. Kiss. Make Love. Repeat.
- Forgive yourself
- And... see it all as a Restart!